PAIN FREE

PERIOD

Comprehensive guide to proven natural remedies and holistic solutions

Dedicated to my daughter, and all the women, in the hope that your journey through womanhood is embraced with comfort and strength.

Table of Contents

Introduction: *Discover Natural and Holistic Solutions for Menstrual Pain Relief*

Welcome to a world where menstrual pain no longer dominates your life. In this book, we will embark on a journey to explore all-natural and holistic treatments and remedies that provide immediate pain relief, as well as address the long-term effects and prevention of menstrual discomfort. For countless women, menstruation is accompanied by bouts of agonizing pain, leaving them feeling helpless and robbed of their vitality. The conventional approach often involves reaching for painkillers, which only offer temporary relief while neglecting the underlying causes of the pain. There are also short term or long term side effects to medications, which someone can not or doesn't want to tolerate. But what if there was a different path to follow? What if there were natural alternatives that could alleviate your pain and promote balance within your body?

When it comes to finding relief from menstrual pain, it's natural to search for remedies that actually work.

This book is a comprehensive guide, carefully crafted to equip you with knowledge and tools to combat menstrual pain the all-natural way. From traditional remedies passed down through generations to cutting-edge holistic treatments backed by scientific research, we have gathered the most effective strategies that have been proven to provide relief and support your overall well-being.

Researchers have found that some herbs contain compounds that possess anti-inflammatory and analgesic properties, which can help to reduce pain and inflammation associated with menstruation. These studies indicate that incorporating herbal remedies into your menstrual pain management routine could be worth considering.

Some research have been done on other medication alternatives like supplements, as well as on techniques like exercise, yoga, and such. We summoned all those were there was some proof they worked.

While scientific studies provide valuable insights, personal experiences and testimonials can also shed light on the effectiveness of different remedies. Many women have reported positive results after using herbs for menstrual pain relief. Some have even described it as a "game-changer" in their monthly battle against discomfort.

Of course, everyone's body is unique, and what works for one person may not work for another. However, the abundance of positive experiences shared by women who have tried alternative remedies suggests that it may be worth a try if you're seeking natural relief from menstrual pain.

Within these pages, you will find detailed information, step-by-step instructions, and advice on various natural and holistic approaches.

Immediate pain relief is just the tip of the iceberg. We delve deeper into the long-term effects of menstrual pain, recognizing the toll it can take on your daily life and overall health.

Understanding menstrual pain, processes involved, and what do we need to address to manage it

Menstrual pain, also known as dysmenorrhea, is a common phenomenon experienced by many menstruating individuals. The pain is typically associated with the menstrual cycle and occurs in the pelvic area. The mechanisms underlying menstrual pain are multifaceted, involving hormonal changes, inflammation, and the role of certain substances like vasopressin.

- ✓ Hormonal Changes:
  - ○ *Prostaglandins: One of the primary contributors to menstrual pain is an increase in the levels of prostaglandins. Prostaglandins are hormone-like substances that play a crucial role in various bodily functions, including the regulation of inflammation and pain. During menstruation, the uterus produces higher levels of prostaglandins, leading to increased uterine contractions. Shrinking blood vessels carry less oxygen rich blood, which means less oxygen getting to the uterus.*

- These contractions are necessary for shedding the uterine lining but can cause pain when they are too strong or prolonged.
  - *Estrogen and Progesterone*: Hormonal changes throughout the menstrual cycle, particularly fluctuations in estrogen and progesterone levels, also contribute to menstrual pain. In the days leading up to menstruation, there is a decrease in progesterone levels, which can trigger inflammation and muscle contractions.

✓ **Inflammation:**

  - *Cytokines and Inflammatory Mediators*: In response to hormonal fluctuations and tissue damage during menstruation, the body's immune system releases various inflammatory mediators, including cytokines. These substances contribute to the inflammatory response, leading to localized swelling, pain, and increased sensitivity to pain.
  - *Leukotrienes*: Prostaglandins and leukotrienes, both derived from arachidonic acid, are lipid mediators involved in the inflammatory response. They promote smooth muscle contraction, enhance pain sensitivity, and contribute to the overall inflammatory cascade associated with menstrual pain.

✓ **Role of Vasopressin:**

- *Vasopressin and Uterine Contractions: Vasopressin, also known as antidiuretic hormone (ADH), is a hormone produced by the hypothalamus and released by the pituitary gland. It plays a role in regulating water balance in the body and constricting blood vessels. During menstruation, elevated levels of vasopressin may contribute to increased uterine contractions and muscle spasms, intensifying menstrual pain.*
  - *Vasopressin and Pain Sensitivity: Vasopressin has been associated with increased pain sensitivity. High levels of vasopressin may enhance the perception of pain, making individuals more prone to experiencing intense menstrual cramps.*

Understanding the interplay of these hormonal and inflammatory factors provides insight into the mechanisms that contribute to menstrual pain. While these processes are essential for the normal functioning of the reproductive system, an imbalance or heightened response can lead to excessive pain and discomfort during menstruation. Management of menstrual pain often involves addressing these mechanisms. Nonsteroidal anti-inflammatory drugs (NSAIDs) are commonly used to reduce prostaglandin production and alleviate inflammation. Hormonal contraceptives, such as birth control pills, can help regulate hormonal fluctuations and reduce the severity of menstrual pain. Lifestyle modifications, such as heat therapy and regular exercise, can also provide relief by promoting muscle relaxation and reducing inflammation.

It's important for individuals experiencing severe or persistent menstrual pain to consult with a healthcare professional for a comprehensive evaluation and tailored treatment plan.

Treating Menstrual Pain Naturally: Exploring Herbal Preparations

Menstrual pain, also known as dysmenorrhea, affects many women worldwide. It can range from mild discomfort to severe cramping, disrupting daily activities and overall well-being. While over-the-counter pain relievers are commonly used, some women prefer natural alternatives. In recent years, several herbal preparations have gained attention for their potential in alleviating menstrual pain. In this book, we will explore the benefits of fennel, california poppy, cinnamon, pycnogenol, bromelain, parsley seed extract, apium seed extract, and many other herbal remedies in treating menstrual pain. Their advantage lies not only in their effectiveness but also in their favorable safety profiles and minimal side effects compared to NSAID medications.

Fennel (Foeniculum vulgare)

Fennel (Foeniculum vulgare) is a medicinal herb that has been used for centuries to address various health issues, including menstrual pain. Rich in volatile oils, such as anethole, fenchone, and estragole, fennel possesses antispasmodic, analgesic, and anti-inflammatory properties that can help alleviate cramping and reduce pain.

Dosage and Preparation

There are different ways to incorporate fennel into your menstrual pain treatment regime. Here are a few dosage and preparation methods:

- **Fennel Tea:** *Steep 1 teaspoon of crushed fennel seeds in 1 cup of boiling water for 10-15 minutes. Strain and drink this soothing tea up to three times a day during your menstrual cycle.*
- **Fennel Capsules:** *Take 400-600 mg of fennel seed capsules up to three times a day. Ensure that the capsules are made from organic fennel seeds to ensure maximum therapeutic benefits.*
- **Fennel Essential Oil:** *Dilute a few drops of fennel essential oil in a carrier oil, such as coconut or jojoba oil, and massage it onto your lower abdomen. Be sure to patch test the oil before applying it to the skin.*

Synergistic Herbs

While fennel can work wonders on its own, combining it with other herbs can enhance its effectiveness and provide a synergistic healing effect. Here are a few herbs that work well in combination with fennel:

- ❖ *Ginger root (Zingiber officinale): Known for its anti-inflammatory and pain-relieving properties, ginger can be consumed as a tea, added to meals, or taken in supplement form. Combining ginger with fennel can promote better pain relief and reduce menstrual cramps.*

- ❖ *Chamomile (Matricaria chamomilla): This gentle herb is often used for its calming and antispasmodic properties. Drinking chamomile tea alongside fennel can help relax the uterus, ease cramps, and reduce discomfort.*

- ❖ *Dong Quai (Angelica sinensis): This traditional Chinese herb is known for its ability to regulate menstrual cycles and reduce pain. Combining it with fennel can offer comprehensive relief by reducing both intensity and duration of menstrual pain.*

Precautions and Considerations

While fennel and other synergistic herbs are generally safe for most individuals, it's important to consider the following precautions:

If you're pregnant or breastfeeding, avoid consuming fennel or other herbal remedies without proper medical advice.

Always use high-quality herbs from trusted sources to ensure their safety and effectiveness.

If menstrual pain persists or worsens, seek medical attention to rule out any underlying conditions.

> *Consult with a healthcare professional before using herbal remedies, especially if you have any existing medical conditions or are taking medications.*

Incorporating fennel into your treatment regime, whether through tea, capsules, or essential oil, can be highly beneficial. Combining it with other herbs can provide enhanced pain-relieving effects.

California Poppy (Eschscholzia californica)

California poppy is a gentle sedative and analgesic herb known for its pain-relieving properties. It can calm the nervous system and help alleviate menstrual cramps.

Preparations and Dosage

California Poppy can be prepared in various ways to effectively tackle menstrual pain. Finding the right dosage for menstrual pain may require some trial and error. Start with a low dose and gradually increase until you find the dosage that works for you. Here are some preparations you can try:

- ❖ Tincture: *A tincture is a concentrated liquid extract of the herb. To make a California Poppy tincture, fill a glass jar with dried California Poppy herb, cover it with a high-proof alcohol like vodka or brandy, and let it sit for four to six weeks. Strain the liquid and store it in a dark glass bottle. Tinctures are taken in small dropperfuls, usually mixed with water or juice.Take 1-2 dropperfuls (about 30-60 drops) up to three times daily as needed*

- ❖ Tea: *California Poppy tea can be made by boiling 1-2 teaspoons of dried herb in a cup of water for 10-15 minutes. Allow the tea to cool, strain it, and drink it throughout the day as needed. Drink 1-2 cups of California Poppy tea per day, as needed.*

- ❖ **Capsules**: *California Poppy capsules can be found in health food stores or prepared at home using powdered or finely ground dried herb. Fill empty capsules with the powder and consume as directed. Follow the instructions on the packaging or consult with a qualified herbalist for proper dosage.*

Possible Synergic Herbs

Combining California Poppy with other herbs may enhance its effectiveness in treating menstrual pain. Here are some herbs that may synergize well:

- ❖ *Cramp Bark (Viburnum opulus): Known for its antispasmodic properties, cramp bark can help relax the muscles and alleviate cramping associated with menstrual pain. It can be taken in tincture or tea form.*
- ❖ *Ginger (Zingiber officinale): Ginger has anti-inflammatory properties that can help reduce pain and inflammation associated with menstrual pain. Consume ginger tea or add fresh ginger to your meals.*
- ❖ *Black Cohosh (Actaea racemosa): This herb has been traditionally used to relieve menstrual pain. It can be taken in tincture or capsule form.*
- ❖ *Chamomile (Matricaria chamomilla): Chamomile has calming properties and can help reduce overall discomfort and pain. Take it in tea form.*

Experiment with different preparations and dosages to find what works best for you. If desired, consider combining it with other synergic herbs to enhance its effects. However, ensure that you consult with a professional for personalized advice that takes your specific health needs into accont.

Cinnamon (Cinnamomum verum)

Cinnamon has been traditionally used to soothe menstrual pain. It contains compounds that possess anti-inflammatory and antispasmodic effects, providing relief from cramping. While it may not work for everyone, it is worth exploring as a natural remedy. Here is some information on preparations, dosage, and possible synergic herbs to consider:

Preparations and Dosage

- ❖ **Tea:** *Boil a teaspoon of cinnamon powder or a cinnamon stick in a cup of water for 10 minutes. Let it cool, strain, and drink. Cinnamon Tea: Drink 1-2 cups of cinnamon tea per day, starting a day or two before your menstrual cycle and continuing until the pain subsides.*

- ❖ **Capsules:** *Take cinnamon capsules that are specifically made for medicinal purposes. Follow the dosage instructions provided on the packaging. Cinnamon Capsules: Follow the recommended dosage mentioned on the packaging. It is usually between 500 mg to 2000 mg per day.*

Possible Synergic Herbs

- ❖ **Ginger:** *Known for its anti-inflammatory properties, ginger can help relieve menstrual pain. You can add* *fresh ginger slices to your cinnamon tea or consume ginger capsules.*

- ❖ **Chamomile:** *Chamomile tea has calming effects and can help reduce cramps. Combining it with cinnamon tea may provide additional relief.*
- ❖ **Turmeric:** *Turmeric contains curcumin, a compound with anti-inflammatory properties. Mixing a pinch of turmeric powder with cinnamon tea could enhance its effectiveness.*

Please note that while cinnamon is generally considered safe, some people may be allergic or sensitive to it. If you experience any adverse reactions or if your symptoms worsen, it is advisable to consult a healthcare professional.

French Maritime Pine extract - Pycnogenol

Derived from the bark of French maritime pine (Pinus pinaster) trees, pycnogenol is a powerful antioxidant and anti-inflammatory agent. Research suggests that pycnogenol can reduce menstrual pain and improve overall well-being during menstrual periods.

Dosage and Preparations

- *The appropriate **dosage** of Pycnogenol for menstrual pain varies, and it is advisable to consult with a healthcare professional before starting any new supplement regimen. However, several studies suggest a standard dosage of 30-60 mg per day.*
- *Pycnogenol is available in various forms, including capsules, tablets, and powders. Capsules and tablets are the most common and convenient forms for consumption. When selecting a Pycnogenol supplement, ensure that it is standardized to contain a sufficient amount of active ingredients.*

Potential Synergic Herbs

Combining Pycnogenol with other herbs can enhance its effectiveness in treating menstrual pain. Here are a few potential herbs that may offer synergistic benefits:

- ❖ *Ginger: Known for its anti-inflammatory and analgesic properties, ginger can complement the effects of Pycnogenol in relieving menstrual pain. It can be consumed as a tea or added to dishes for its flavor and medicinal benefits.*
- ❖ *Turmeric: Curcumin, the active compound in turmeric, possesses potent anti-inflammatory properties. When combined with Pycnogenol, it can provide additional pain relief. Turmeric can be added to meals or taken as a supplement.*
- ❖ *Cramp Bark: As the name suggests, cramp bark has been traditionally used to alleviate menstrual cramps. When used alongside Pycnogenol, it may help reduce pain intensity and duration. Cramp bark is available in various forms such as capsules, tinctures, or teas.*
- ❖ *Chamomile: Chamomile is a well-known herb with calming and anti-inflammatory properties. Consuming chamomile tea along with Pycnogenol can help relax the muscles and reduce menstrual pain.*

Precautions and Considerations

While Pycnogenol is generally safe for most individuals, it is important to exercise caution and consider the following points:

Always consult with a healthcare professional before starting any new supplement regimen, especially if you have any underlying health conditions or if you are on medication.

Pregnant or breastfeeding women should avoid using Pycnogenol unless advised by a qualified healthcare professional.

Some individuals may experience mild side effects such as gastrointestinal discomfort or headaches. If these symptoms persist, consider adjusting the dosage or discontinuing use.

Pycnogenol may interact with certain medications, including blood thinners. It is important to inform your healthcare provider about any supplements you are taking to avoid any potential drug interactions.

Pineapple extract –Bromelain

Bromelain is extracted from the stems and fruit of pineapple plants. Its anti-inflammatory and pain-relieving properties have made it a popular supplement for various conditions. It helps reduce menstrual pain by decreasing prostaglandin levels, which are responsible for triggering uterine contractions and subsequent pain during menstruation.

Dosage and Preparations

Bromelain supplements are available in various forms, including capsules, tablets, and powders. They can be found in health stores and online retailers. It is important to choose a reputable brand that offers pure bromelain without any harmful additives.

When using bromelain for the management of menstrual pain, dosage is essential. The appropriate dosage can vary depending on the strength of the bromelain supplement. However, it is generally recommended to start with a low dosage and gradually increase if necessary. The following guidelines can help:

- ❖ **Low/Standard Dosage:** *400-800 milligrams (mg) of bromelain per day, spread across multiple doses.*
- ❖ **High Dosage:** *Not exceeding 2000mg of bromelain per day.*

It is crucial to follow the instructions provided on the specific product label or consult with a healthcare professional to determine the appropriate dosage for individual needs.

Potential Synergistic Herbs:

While bromelain can provide relief from menstrual pain on its own, combining it with other synergistic herbs may enhance its effectiveness. Below are a few herbs that you may consider incorporating with bromelain:

- ❖ *Ginger: Ginger has long been used as a natural remedy for menstrual pain due to its anti-inflammatory and analgesic properties. Combining bromelain with ginger can provide a potent anti-pain effect.*
- ❖ *Turmeric: With its active compound curcumin, turmeric also possesses anti-inflammatory properties. Pairing bromelain with turmeric can result in a more robust anti-pain synergy.*
- ❖ *Cramp Bark: This herb's name says it all. Cramp bark has antispasmodic properties and is commonly used to relieve menstrual cramps. Bromelain and cramp bark can work together to provide relief from both pain and spasms.*
- ❖ *Chamomile: Known for its calming effects, chamomile can help reduce stress and relax the muscles. When combined with bromelain, it can contribute to overall pain relief during menstruation.*

Parsley Seed Extract

Parsley seed extract is derived from the seeds of the parsley plant (Petroselinum crispum). It contains various bioactive compounds, including volatile oils, flavonoids, and antioxidants, which contribute to its therapeutic benefits. These compounds possess anti-inflammatory properties that can help reduce the pain associated with menstrual cramps. Parsley seed extract is known for its diuretic properties, helping to eliminate excess water retention and reduce bloating during menstruation.

Dosage and Preparations

Parsley seed extract is readily available in health stores and online retailers. Look for products that contain standardized amounts of the active compounds. It is advisable to consult product labels or seek guidance from healthcare professionals for accurate usage instructions and potential contraindications

When using parsley seed extract to address menstrual pain, determining the appropriate dosage is essential for optimal results. Although there is no standardized dosage for parsley seed extract specifically for menstrual pain, the following general guidelines can be useful:

- ❖ **Low/Standard Dosage:** *Start with 250-500 milligrams (mg) of parsley seed extract per day, taken orally. It is* *recommended to split the dosage into two or three administrations throughout the day.*

- ❖ **High Dosage:** *If necessary, the dosage can be increased gradually up to 1000mg per day. However, it is always advisable to consult with a healthcare professional before using higher doses.*

It is crucial to choose a reputable brand that provides pure and potent parsley seed extract in the form of capsules or tinctures for easier and accurate dosage administration.

Potential Synergistic Herbs:

While parsley seed extract can be effective on its own, combining it with synergistic herbs may augment its benefits for alleviating menstrual pain. Consider the following herbal options:

- ❖ *Cramp Bark: Known for its antispasmodic properties, cramp bark can help reduce muscle spasms and ease menstrual cramps. Combining parsley seed extract with cramp bark may provide a more comprehensive approach to alleviating pain.*

- ❖ *Ginger: Ginger has anti-inflammatory and pain-relieving properties, which can complement the effects of parsley seed extract. It may help further reduce inflammation and ease menstrual pain.*

- ❖ *Chamomile: Chamomile possesses soothing and calming properties. When combined with parsley seed* extract, it can contribute to reducing stress and improving overall well-being during menstruation.

❖ *Valerian Root:* Valerian root has sedative properties and may aid in relaxation. Its combination with parsley seed extract may help alleviate pain and promote restful sleep during menstruation.

Apium Seed Extract

While there are various remedies available, one lesser-known option is apium seed extract. Apium seed extract is derived from celery seeds (Apium graveolens) and has been traditionally used for its analgesic and anti-inflammatory properties. It is believed to work by promoting blood flow and reducing inflammation.

Preparations of Apium Seed Extract

Apium seed extract can be found in various forms, including capsules, tinctures, powders, and teas. Choosing the most suitable preparation depends on individual preferences and the desired convenience.

- ❖ **Capsules:** Apium seed extract capsules are a common and convenient option. They provide a standardized dosage and can be easily taken with water.
- ❖ **Tinctures:** Tinctures are liquid extracts made by soaking apium seeds in alcohol or a solvent. They offer a fast-absorbing option, and the dosage can be easily adjusted by adding or reducing drops.
- ❖ **Powders:** Apium seed extract powders can be added to smoothies, juices, or other beverages. This form allows for creative integration with other herbal remedies to enhance their effectiveness.
- ❖ **Teas:** While less concentrated than extracts, apium seed teas can be a soothing and comforting option.

Boiling apium seeds in water and steeping for several minutes can yield a homemade tea.

Dosage of Apium Seed Extract

When using apium seed extract for menstrual pain relief, it is crucial to follow the recommended dosage guidelines. The optimal dosage may vary depending on factors such as the severity of pain and individual response.Typically, a starting point would be to take 500 mg of apium seed extract capsules, one to three times daily. However, the dosage can be adjusted based on the individual's needs and response. It is important to note that exceeding the recommended dosage may lead to unwanted side effects and should be avoided.

Possible Synergistic Herbs

To maximize the benefits of apium seed extract for menstrual pain relief, it can be combined with other synergistic herbs. The following herbs are known for their analgesic, antispasmodic, and hormone-balancing properties:

- ❖ *Chamomile: Chamomile has anti-inflammatory properties, calming effects, and can help relieve muscle spasms. When combined with apium seed extract, it may enhance the pain-relieving effects.*
- ❖ *Ginger: Ginger has been used for centuries to alleviate pain and reduce inflammation. It can be combined with apium seed extract to help ease menstrual cramps and provide overall relief.*

- ❖ *Cramp Bark: Cramp bark (Viburnum opulus) is widely known for its ability to relax the smooth muscles of the uterus. Combining cramp bark with apium seed extract can provide synergistic relief for menstrual pain.*
- ❖ *Black Cohosh: Black Cohosh is a herb known for its hormonal balancing effects and potential pain relief. When combined with apium seed extract, it can help regulate hormonal imbalances that contribute to menstrual pain.*

Before combining any herbs, it is essential to consult a healthcare professional or herbalist to ensure they are safe and compatible for individual use. The dosages and preparations of these synergistic herbs may vary, and expert guidance is beneficial.

Cramp Bark and its Benefits

Cramp bark, scientifically known as Viburnum opulus, has been traditionally used for centuries to alleviate menstrual cramps. It is believed to work by relaxing the uterine muscles and reducing inflammation, ultimately relieving pain associated with menstrual cramps.

Dosage and Preparations:

When using cramp bark to treat menstrual cramps, it is crucial to consult with a healthcare professional to determine the appropriate dosage. However, here are some general guidelines:

- ❖ *Tea: One common way to consume cramp bark is by brewing it into a tea. To prepare the tea, add 1-2 teaspoons of dried cramp bark to a cup of boiling water. Let it steep for about 10-15 minutes before straining. Drinking this tea two to three times a day during the menstrual cycle may help alleviate cramp pain.*

- ❖ *Capsules or Tinctures: Cramp bark is also available in capsule or tincture form. Cramp bark tincture may provide quick relief for menstrual pain and help relax the muscles, reducing cramping. It is believed to work by blocking nerve signals that trigger excessive muscle contractions. Follow the instructions provided by the manufacturer or consult a healthcare professional for the recommended dosage for your specific needs.*

- ❖ **Dosage**: *Cramp bark tinctures are concentrated liquid extracts. Follow the manufacturer's instructions for dosage recommendations. Typically, 1-2 mL (approximately 30-60 drops) diluted in water, three times a day, is a common dosage. Consult a herbalist or healthcare professional for personalized dosing guidance.*

It's important to note that individual responses to cramp bark may vary, so it's essential to start with smaller doses and gradually increase if necessary.

Synergic Herbs to Enhance Effectiveness:

Cramp bark can be combined with other herbs to maximize its effectiveness in relieving menstrual cramps. Some potential synergic herbs include:

- ❖ *Ginger: Known for its anti-inflammatory properties, ginger may help reduce pain and inflammation associated with menstrual cramps. You can add ginger to your cramp bark tea or consume it separately.*
- ❖ *Chamomile: Chamomile has calming properties that can help relax muscles and relieve menstrual cramp pain. Infuse chamomile flowers along with cramp bark when brewing your tea for added benefits.*
- ❖ *Black Cohosh: This herb is often used to alleviate symptoms of menopause, but it may also help reduce*

menstrual cramp severity. Combining black cohosh with cramp bark can offer enhanced relief.

Before combining cramp bark with other herbs, it's advisable to consult a healthcare professional or herbalist to ensure compatibility and optimal dosage.

Black Cohosh and its Benefits

Black cohosh, scientifically known as Actaea racemosa, is a herb that has been traditionally used to address various reproductive issues, including menstrual cramps. It is believed to work by promoting muscle relaxation and reducing inflammation, ultimately providing relief from the pain and discomfort associated with menstrual cramps.

Dosage and Preparations:

Dosage guidelines for black cohosh may vary depending on individual needs and health conditions. It's crucial to consult with a healthcare professional or herbalist to determine the appropriate dosage. However, here are some general recommendations:

- ❖ **Standardized Extract:** *Black cohosh is commonly available in the form of standardized extracts, typically containing 1-2 mg of the active ingredient (such as triterpene glycosides) per dose. Follow the instructions provided by the manufacturer or consult a healthcare professional for the recommended dosage.*
- ❖ **Tea Infusion:** *Though less common, black cohosh can also be prepared as a tea infusion. Add 1-2 teaspoons of dried black cohosh root or powder to a cup of boiling water. Let it steep for about 10-15 minutes before straining. Drinking this tea two to three times a*

day during the menstrual cycle may help alleviate cramp pain.

Again, it is important to note that individual responses to black cohosh may vary, so it is wise to start with smaller doses and gradually increase if needed, under the guidance of a healthcare professional.

Synergic Herbs to Enhance Effectiveness:
Combining black cohosh with other herbs may enhance its effectiveness in relieving menstrual cramps. Here are a few potential synergistic herbs:

- ❖ *Cramp Bark: Cramp bark is known for its muscle-relaxing properties and can complement the effects of black cohosh. It can be brewed into a tea along with black cohosh or taken in other forms.*
- ❖ *Ginger: Ginger possesses anti-inflammatory properties and may help reduce pain and inflammation associated with menstrual cramps. Combine ginger with black cohosh by adding it to tea or consuming it separately.*
- ❖ *Red Raspberry Leaf: Red raspberry leaf is commonly used to tone the uterus and relieve menstrual cramps. It can be added to the black cohosh tea for added benefits.*

As with any herbal combination, it is always advisable to consult a healthcare professional or herbalist to ensure compatibility, appropriate dosages, and any potential contraindications.

Turmeric for Menstrual Cramps

Turmeric, scientifically known as Curcuma longa, has been used for centuries in traditional medicine for its anti-inflammatory and pain-relieving properties. One of the active compounds in turmeric, called curcumin, has shown promise in reducing pain and inflammation associated with menstrual cramps.

Curcumin, the active compound in turmeric, has demonstrated promising anti-inflammatory and analgesic properties. Studies have found curcumin to be effective in reducing both pain intensity and duration of menstrual pain. Its potential as a natural alternative is further supported by its excellent safety profile.

Preparations of Turmeric

There are various ways to incorporate turmeric into your routine to manage menstrual cramps:

- ❖ **Tea:** *Brew a teaspoon of turmeric powder in a cup of hot water. Add honey or lemon for flavor.*
- ❖ **Capsules or Supplements:** *Available in most health stores, these supplements provide a standardized dosage of curcumin.*
- ❖ **Golden Milk:** *Mix one teaspoon of turmeric powder with warm milk, a pinch of black pepper, and some honey or cinnamon. This soothing drink can be consumed before bed or during the day for pain relief.*

- ❖ **Turmeric Massage Oil:** *Massage painful areas with a mixture of turmeric powder and a carrier oil, such as coconut or jojoba oil. This can help alleviate both the pain and inflammation associated with menstrual cramps.*

Dosage Recommendations

When using turmeric for menstrual cramps, it is crucial to ensure the correct dosage to achieve optimal results. It is generally recommended to take 500 mg to 1,000 mg of turmeric powder, or 50 mg to 100 mg of curcumin extract, three times a day. However, it's important to consult with a healthcare professional or naturopath before starting any supplement regimen, as individual needs may vary.

Possible Synergistic Herbs

While turmeric can be effective on its own, combining it with other herbs may enhance its pain-relieving properties. Some possible synergistic herbs that can be used in conjunction with turmeric for menstrual cramps include:

- ❖ *Ginger: Like turmeric, ginger possesses anti-inflammatory properties and may help alleviate menstrual cramps. Consuming ginger tea or adding ginger to your diet may provide additional relief.*
- ❖ *Cinnamon: This warming spice has anti-inflammatory properties that can help reduce pain. Try adding*

cinnamon to turmeric golden milk or other warm beverages.

- ❖ *Chamomile: Known for its calming and antispasmodic properties, chamomile tea may help relax the uterine muscles and reduce menstrual cramp discomfort.*
- ❖ *Black Cohosh: Primarily used for menopause symptoms, black cohosh may help regulate and lessen menstrual cramp intensity.*

Remember, it is essential to consult with a healthcare professional or naturopath before combining herbs or starting any new supplement routine, especially if you have any underlying health conditions or are taking medications.

Boswellia for Menstrual Cramps

Boswellia is a resin derived from the Boswellia serrata tree, native to India. It contains compounds that have anti-inflammatory and analgesic properties, making it an effective supplement for reducing inflammation and pain. Menstrual cramps are caused by the contraction of the uterine muscles, and boswellia can help to relax these muscles and reduce the associated pain. Additionally, the anti-inflammatory properties of boswellia can reduce inflammation in the pelvic area, further reducing cramping and discomfort.

Dosage and Preparations

The recommended dosage of boswellia for menstrual cramps varies depending on the individual and the severity of their symptoms. Typical dosages range from 300-500mg of boswellia extract daily, but it is important to consult with a healthcare professional before starting a new supplement regimen. Boswellia can be taken in capsules, tablets, or as a liquid extract, and should be taken with a meal to aid in absorption.

Potential Synergistic Herbs

While boswellia can be effective on its own for treating menstrual cramps, it can be even more effective when combined with other herbs that have complementary properties. One such herb is ginger, which also has anti-inflammatory properties and can help to reduce nausea associated with menstrual cramps. Another herb that can be beneficial is cramp bark, which has been traditionally used to reduce muscle spasms and cramping. When taken in recommended doses and in combination with other synergistic herbs, it can be an even more effective treatment option. As with any supplement, it is important to consult with a healthcare professional before starting a new regimen.

Ginger for Menstrual Pain Relief

Ginger, a well-known herbal remedy, has been found to be as effective as NSAIDs in reducing menstrual pain. Several studies have shown that ginger's anti-inflammatory properties can significantly alleviate dysmenorrhea. Additionally, ginger has a favorable safety profile and lacks the potential side effects associated with NSAID use. Its efficacy and safety make ginger a promising alternative to consider for menstrual pain relief.

Ginger possesses natural anti-inflammatory and analgesic properties, making it a valuable herb for relieving menstrual pain. Its active compound, gingerol, is known to inhibit pain-causing chemicals in the body, thus reducing the intensity of menstrual cramps and discomfort.

Moreover, ginger has been found to suppress the production of prostaglandins, hormone-like substances that contribute to uterine contractions and pain during menstruation. By alleviating prostaglandin levels, ginger helps to ease the severity of menstrual pain.

Preparations and Dosage

- ❖ *Ginger Tea: One of the simplest and most popular ways to consume ginger is by preparing ginger tea. To make ginger tea, follow these steps:*
    - ○ *Take a 1-inch piece of fresh ginger root and peel off the skin.*
    - ○ *Slice the ginger into thin pieces or grate it.*

- o   *Boil 2 cups of water and add the ginger.*
- o   *Simmer for 10-15 minutes.*
- o   *Strain the tea and add a natural sweetener like honey if desired.*
- o   *Drink this tea 2-3 times a day during your menstrual period.*

❖ **Ginger Capsules**: *Ginger capsules are a convenient option for those who prefer not to consume ginger directly. You can find ginger capsules or supplements in health food stores or pharmacies. Follow the recommended dosage instructions provided by the manufacturer or consult a healthcare professional for guidance.*

❖ **Fresh Ginger**: *If you prefer consuming fresh ginger, you can add it to your meals or incorporate it into smoothies or juices. Start with a 1-inch piece of grated ginger and gradually increase the quantity according to your tolerance and effectiveness.*

❖ **Ginger Oil**: *Another way to use ginger is by applying ginger oil topically. Mix a few drops of ginger essential oil with a carrier oil like coconut oil, and massage it onto your lower abdomen. This can provide localized relief from menstrual pain.*

Possible Synergic Herbs

While ginger alone can be effective in relieving menstrual pain, combining it with other herbs may enhance its pain-relieving properties. Some synergistic herbs that can be used alongside ginger include:

- ❖ **Turmeric:** *Turmeric contains curcumin, a powerful anti-inflammatory compound. Combining turmeric with ginger can provide potent pain relief due to their complementary anti-inflammatory effects.*
- ❖ **Cinnamon:** *Cinnamon has been shown to possess analgesic properties and can help alleviate menstrual pain when used in conjunction with ginger. Add a pinch of cinnamon to your ginger tea or include it in your meals for added benefits.*
- ❖ **Chamomile:** *Chamomile is known for its calming and relaxing properties. Combining chamomile with ginger can not only help ease menstrual pain but also help reduce stress and promote better sleep.*

Precautions and Conclusion

Though ginger is generally safe for consumption, it is essential to consider a few precautions. Pregnant women, individuals with blood clotting disorders, or those taking blood-thinning medications should consult their healthcare provider before using ginger or any other herbal remedy.

Chamomile for Menstrual Pain Relief

Chamomile is a herb that belongs to the daisy family and is known for its calming and anti-inflammatory properties. It contains flavonoids, which have anti-spasmodic effects that help to ease uterine contractions, thus reducing menstrual pain. Chamomile is also an effective natural remedy for reducing inflammation and swelling of the uterus, further minimizing menstrual pain.

Preparations and Dosage

- ❖ *Tea: One of the most common ways to consume chamomile is by preparing chamomile tea. To make chamomile tea, follow these simple steps:*
    - ○ *Boil a cup of water.*
    - ○ *Add 2-3 teaspoons of dried chamomile flowers or one chamomile tea bag to the boiling water.*
    - ○ *Cover and let steep for 5-10 minutes.*
    - ○ *Strain the tea and add a natural sweetener such as honey or lemon if desired.*
    - ○ *Drink 2-3 cups of chamomile tea per day during your menstrual cycle.*
- ❖ *Tincture: Chamomile tincture is another option for consuming chamomile. A tincture is a concentrated herbal extract made by soaking chamomile flowers in alcohol for several weeks. Dosage recommendations vary, but it is best to follow the instructions*

recommended by the manufacturer or consult a healthcare professional.

❖ **Chamomile Essential Oil:** *Chamomile essential oil is a concentrated oil obtained from chamomile flowers. It can be applied topically or added to a warm bath to help alleviate menstrual pain. Mix a few drops of chamomile essential oil with a carrier oil like almond or coconut oil before applying it to the lower abdomen.*

❖ **Capsules:** *Chamomile capsules are also available, but it is essential to follow the recommended dosage guidelines provided on the bottle or consult with a healthcare professional before use.*

Possible Synergic Herbs

While chamomile can help alleviate menstrual pain on its own, combining it with other herbs can enhance its pain-relieving properties.

❖ **Ginger:** *Ginger is well known for its anti-inflammatory and analgesic properties. Combining chamomile with ginger can help alleviate menstrual pain and cramps by reducing inflammation and easing uterine contractions.*

❖ **Cinnamon:** *Cinnamon has anti-inflammatory and analgesic properties that can provide relief from menstrual pain. Drinking cinnamon tea alongside* *chamomile tea can help reduce menstrual pain and cramps.*

- ❖ **Valerian Root:** *Valerian root is known for its calming and sedative properties. It can help reduce stress and anxiety, which can contribute to menstrual pain. Combining chamomile with valerian root can provide pain relief and promote relaxation.*

Precautions and Conclusion

While chamomile is safe for consumption, some individuals may experience side effects such as allergic reactions or drowsiness. It is important to consult with a healthcare professional before using chamomile or any other herbal remedies, especially if you are on medication or have underlying health conditions.

Treating Menstrual Pain with Paeony Root

Paeony root is derived from the peony plant (Paeonia lactiflora) and has been used in traditional Chinese medicine for centuries. It is prized for its anti-inflammatory, analgesic, and muscle-relaxing properties, which make it an excellent natural remedy for menstrual pain. Paeony root contains active compounds such as paeoniflorin and albiflorin, which alleviate pain and reduce inflammation.

Preparations of Paeony Root

Paeony root can be found in various forms, including dried root slices, powders, tinctures, and capsules. Here are a few common preparations:

- ❖ *Dried Root Slices: These can be brewed into a tea by simmering 1-2 teaspoons of dried root slices in a cup of water for 15-20 minutes. The tea can be consumed up to three times a day, starting a few days before the onset of menstrual pain.*
- ❖ *Powders: Paeony root powder can be added to smoothies, soups, or other food preparations. Start with 1-2 grams per day and gradually increase the dosage if necessary. It is advisable to consult a healthcare professional for personalized dosage recommendations.*

- ❖ *Tinctures: Paeony root tinctures are concentrated liquid extracts usually made by soaking the herb in alcohol or glycerin. Follow the manufacturer's instructions or consult a herbalist for the appropriate dosage and usage.*
- ❖ *Capsules: Paeony root is available in capsule form, providing a convenient way to consume the herb. Follow the recommended dosage on the product label or seek guidance from a healthcare professional*

Dosage Recommendations

When it comes to dosing paeony root, it is essential to start with a small amount and gradually increase based on individual response. As an herbal supplement, the appropriate dosage may vary from person to person. As a general guideline, consider the following dosages:

- ❖ *Dried Root Slices: 1-2 teaspoons brewed into a cup of tea, up to three times a day.*
- ❖ *Powders: Start with 1-2 grams per day, increasing gradually if needed.*
- ❖ *Tinctures: Follow the manufacturer's instructions or consult a herbalist for accurate dosage recommendations.*
- ❖ *Capsules: Follow the recommended dosage on the product label or seek guidance from a healthcare professional.*

It is crucial to remember that everyone's body reacts differently to herbal remedies, so finding the right dosage may require some trial and error. If any adverse effects occur, reduce or discontinue use and consult a healthcare professional.

Potential Synergic Herbs

Paeony root can be combined with other herbs to enhance its pain-relieving properties. Here are a few synergistic herbs that may have complementary effects:

- ❖ *Ginger: Known for its anti-inflammatory and analgesic properties, ginger can be added to teas or meals alongside paeony root to relieve menstrual pain.*

- ❖ *Cramp Bark: Cramp bark has been traditionally used for muscle relaxation and menstrual cramp relief. Combining it with paeony root may provide a more comprehensive approach to managing menstrual pain.*

- ❖ *Chamomile: Chamomile has soothing properties that can help reduce menstrual pain and relax muscles. It can be consumed as a tea in combination with paeony root.*

- ❖ *Dong Quai: Often used in traditional Chinese medicine to balance hormones and alleviate menstrual discomfort, dong quai can be paired with paeony root for enhanced benefits.*

It is advisable to consult a healthcare professional or herbalist before combining different herbs to ensure their compatibility and determine appropriate dosages.

Skullcap

Skullcap (Scutellaria lateriflora) is an herb with calming and anti-inflammatory properties that may help alleviate menstrual pain. It is commonly used to promote relaxation and ease muscle tension.

Dosage: *To prepare skullcap tea, steep 1-2 teaspoons of dried skullcap leaves in a cup of hot water for 10-15 minutes. Drink up to three cups per day, starting a few days before your period.*

Benefits: *Skullcap tea may help reduce stress, anxiety, and muscle tension associated with menstrual pain. By promoting relaxation, it may indirectly alleviate discomfort during menstruation.*

Chaste Tree Berry (Vitex agnus-castus)

Chaste tree berry, also known as Vitex, is believed to influence the hormonal balance by acting on the pituitary gland, helping to regulate the menstrual cycle and reduce symptoms like pain.

Dosage: *Capsules or tinctures of chaste tree berry are available. A common dosage is 20-40 mg of a standardized extract daily. It may take several months to see full benefits.*

Wild Lettuce: A Natural Alternative for Menstrual Pain Treatment

Wild lettuce, scientifically known as Lactuca virosa, is an annual flowering plant that belongs to the Asteraceae family. It is native to Europe and has been naturalized in many parts of the world, including North America. Wild lettuce is known for its medicinal properties and has been traditionally used for various purposes.

The analgesic effect of wild lettuce is primarily due to the presence of the compound lactucopicrin. This compound is responsible for relaxing smooth muscles and inhibiting the release of pain-producing substances in the body. Studies have shown that lactucopicrin exhibits anti-inflammatory and pain-relieving properties, making it a potential candidate for treating menstrual cramps.

Preparation and Dosage

To use wild lettuce for menstrual pain, it is important to use the correct preparation and dosage. Here are some recommended methods:

- ❖ *Tea: Prepare a tea by steeping one teaspoon of dried wild lettuce leaves in a cup of hot water for 10-15 minutes. Strain and drink the tea two or three times per day.*

- ❖ **Capsules:** *Take wild lettuce capsules, following the instructions on the packaging. Make sure to consult with a healthcare professional to determine the appropriate dosage for you.*
- ❖ **Extract:** *Prepare a tincture by soaking wild lettuce leaves in a jar of alcohol for several weeks. Take a few drops of the extract, mixed with water or juice, as needed.*
- ❖ **Compress:** *Soak a cloth in warm water mixed with a few drops of wild lettuce extract and apply it as a compress to the affected area.*

Wild lettuce should not be used by women who are pregnant, breastfeeding, or have hormonal imbalances. It should also not be consumed in large quantities by individuals with liver or kidney problems. Certain medications may interact with it, so it is important to be aware of any potential interactions.Some people may have sensitivities or allergies to wild lettuce. It is recommended to use a small amount at first and monitor for any adverse reactions.

Sidebells Wintergreen, as a Natural Remedy for Menstrual Pain

Throughout history, Sidebells Wintergreen (Orthilia secunda) has been valued for its medicinal properties, particularly in relieving menstrual pain. Traditional healers have used it to ease cramps, reduce inflammation, and promote overall well-being during menstruation. Its effectiveness in providing relief for menstrual pain has made it a popular natural remedy for women. This plant contains various active compounds that contribute to its potential therapeutic effects. These include flavonoids, phenolic acids, and tannins. These compounds have been found to possess antioxidant and anti-inflammatory properties. Orthilia secunda, a herb with a funny-sounding name, has been studied for its potential effectiveness in alleviating menstrual pain. Several scientific studies have shown promising results, suggesting that this herb may indeed offer some relief.

Preparations

- ❖ **Tea:** *One common way to use Sidebells Wintergreen for menstrual pain relief is by preparing a tea. To make Orthilia secunda tea, simply steep about 1-2 teaspoons of the dried leaves and stems in boiling water for 10-15 minutes. You can sweeten it with honey or lemon according to your preference. Sip on* *this soothing tea during your menstrual cycle to potentially alleviate pain and discomfort.*

❖ **Capsules or Extracts:** *If you prefer a more convenient option, there are Orthilia secunda capsules or extracts available in the market. These supplements are typically made from dried Sidebells Wintergreen, and provide a concentrated dose of its active compounds.*

Herbal Combinations for Menstrual Pain Management

While Sidebells Wintergreen shows promise on its own, combining it with other herbal remedies can potentially enhance its effectiveness in managing menstrual pain. Herbs such as ginger, chamomile, and cramp bark have been traditionally used for their pain-relieving properties and can complement the benefits of Orthilia secunda.

Precautions

While Sidebells Wintergreen, is generally considered safe for most people, it's important to be aware of potential interactions with medications. If you are taking any prescription medications or have any underlying health conditions, it's advisable to consult with a healthcare professional before incorporating Orthilia secunda into your routine.Certain medications, such as blood thinners or antiplatelet drugs, may have interactions with Orthilia secunda. It's always better to err on the side of caution and seek professional advice to ensure your safety.As with any herbal supplement, there is a possibility of experiencing allergic reactions or adverse effects. While rare, some individuals may be sensitive to Orthilia secunda or its components. If you notice any unusual symptoms or discomfort after using it, discontinue use and consult a healthcare professional.

Jamaican Dogwood: A Natural Remedy to Alleviate Menstrual Pain

Jamaican Dogwood (Piscidia erythrina) is a tropical tree that grows in the Caribbean, parts of Central and South America, and Florida. It has been traditionally used in herbal medicine to alleviate pain and promote slee]. Its effectiveness in reducing menstrual pain is attributed to its ability to relax the muscles and reduce inflammation.

Preparation

Jamaican Dogwood is available in various forms such as teas, tinctures, capsules, and powders. The most common form is the tincture, which is a concentrated liquid extraction of the plant. Jamaican Dogwood is also available in the form of supplements such as capsules.

Dosage

The optimal dosage of Jamaican Dogwood depends on the form of the supplement and the severity of menstrual pain. It's important to consult with a healthcare professional or a qualified herbalist before incorporating Jamaican Dogwood into your diet.

- ❖ *For tinctures, take 1-2 mL (around 20-40 drops) before bedtime for insomnia or 1-2 mL 2-4 times per day for pain relief.*

- ❖ *Jamaican Dogwood* **capsules** *are also available in the market with a standard dose of 300-500 mg per capsule, and it's recommended to take two to three capsules per day after meals.*

Precautions

While Jamaican Dogwood is considered safe when taken in recommended dosages, it's essential to exercise caution, particularly if you're taking other medications or have certain health conditions. Pregnant or breastfeeding women should avoid using Jamaican Dogwood as it may have negative consequences on fetal development.

Jamaican Dogwood may cause drowsiness, so it's advisable to avoid driving or operating heavy machinery after taking this supplement. The supplement may also interact with other medications such as sedatives, anesthetics, and anti-anxiety drugs. Always consult with a healthcare provider before taking any new supplements.

Chinese Herbal Treatments for Menstrual Cramps: A Natural Approach to Alleviating Discomfort

Chinese herbal treatments offer a natural and holistic approach to managing menstrual cramps. Dong Quai, Chinese peony, ginger, and ligusticum are just a few examples of the herbs that have been used for centuries to alleviate pain, promote blood circulation, and reduce inflammation.

Dong Quai (Angelica sinensis)

Dong Quai, also known as "female ginseng," is one of the most widely used herbs in Chinese medicine for women's health. It has been traditionally used to alleviate menstrual pain and regulate the menstrual cycle by promoting blood circulation and reducing spasms.

Dosage: *Dong Quai is commonly taken as a decoction or in capsule form. A typical dosage is 3-15 grams per day in divided doses. However, it is best to consult a qualified practitioner of Chinese medicine for personalized dosing guidance.*

Benefits: *Dong Quai possesses anti-inflammatory and analgesic properties that can help reduce menstrual cramp intensity and duration. It is also believed to harmonize hormonal balance and regulate menstruation.*

Chinese Peony (Paeonia lactiflora)

Chinese peony, also known as Bai Shao, is a herb highly regarded in Chinese medicine for its ability to alleviate menstrual pain and calm the mind. It helps promote blood flow and soothes muscle contractions.

Dosage: Chinese peony is typically consumed in the form of a decoction or as a powdered extract. A typical dosage is 6-12 grams per day. However, as with any herbal remedy, it is best to consult a professional practitioner for individualized recommendations.

Benefits: Chinese peony has antispasmodic and anti-inflammatory properties that can help relax uterine muscles and reduce cramping. It may also have a calming effect, which can be beneficial for individuals experiencing emotional symptoms alongside menstrual cramps.

Ligusticum (Ligusticum chuanxiong)

Ligusticum, also known as Chuan Xiong, is a popular herb in traditional Chinese medicine for pain relief. It helps promote blood circulation, relieve muscle tension, and alleviate menstrual cramps.

Dosage: Ligusticum is commonly taken as a decoction, herbal extract, or in capsule form. The recommended dosage may vary depending on the specific product and individual needs. Consult a qualified practitioner for accurate dosing instructions.

Benefits: *Ligusticum's properties make it effective in relieving pain and reducing muscle tension associated with menstrual cramps. Its ability to promote blood circulation can also help alleviate stagnant energy and reduce pain intensity.*

68

Seeking Professional Guidance

By seeking guidance from a qualified practitioner of Chinese medicine, you can receive personalized recommendations and create an individualized treatment plan to address your specific needs. By incorporating these herbal remedies, you may find relief from menstrual cramps and improve your overall well-being.

South American Herbal Treatments for Menstrual Pain

Effective Remedies and Dosage

South America is known for its rich biodiversity, which has led to the discovery of various plants with potential analgesic and anti-inflammatory properties. In this book, we will explore some South American herbal treatments for menstrual pain, along with recommended dosages.

Maca (Lepidium meyenii):

Maca has been traditionally used in South America to alleviate menstrual symptoms, including pain and cramps. It is believed to balance hormone levels and support the overall well-being of women. The recommended dosage is 1500-3000 mg per day, divided into two or three doses. Maca is available in powder or capsule form and can be consumed with food or mixed into a beverage.

Chamomile (Matricaria chamomilla):

Chamomile is widely recognized for its calming properties and is commonly used to relax muscles, including the uterus. It helps ease menstrual pain and reduces discomfort. To prepare chamomile tea, steep 2-3 teaspoons of dried chamomile flowers in hot water for about 10 minutes. Consume up to three cups per day, especially during the menstrual period.

Damiana (Turnera diffusa):

Damiana is a herb indigenous to South America, commonly used for its mood-enhancing properties. It can help reduce menstrual pain by relaxing the uterine muscles. For menstrual pain relief, it is recommended to infuse 1-2 teaspoons of dried damiana leaves in a cup of hot water and let it steep for 10-15 minutes. Consume up to three cups per day.

Yarrow (Achillea millefolium):

Yarrow is known for its anti-inflammatory and analgesic properties, making it particularly beneficial for menstrual pain relief. To prepare yarrow tea, steep 1-2 teaspoons of dried yarrow flowers in hot water for about 15 minutes. Consume up to three cups per day during the menstrual period.

Cat's Claw (Uncaria tomentosa):

Cat's Claw is a popular South American herb known for its anti-inflammatory properties. It can help alleviate menstrual pain and reduce inflammation in the reproductive system. Recommended dosage is usually 500-1000 mg per day, taken in capsule form. It is advisable to consult with a healthcare professional before using Cat's Claw as it may interact with certain medications.

African Herbal Treatments for Menstrual Pain: Ancient Remedies and Dosage Guidelines

In Africa, traditional medicine has long utilized the healing properties of various herbs to alleviate menstrual pain. These natural remedies offer an alternative approach for women seeking relief from cramps and discomfort. In this book, we will explore some African herbal treatments for menstrual pain, along with recommended dosages to help women find relief.

Dill (Anethum graveolens):

Dill is another African herb that has been used traditionally to alleviate menstrual pain. It has antispasmodic properties that help relieve muscle cramps. To prepare dill tea, add 2 teaspoons of dried dill seeds or 1 tablespoon of fresh dill to a cup of hot water. Let it steep for 10-15 minutes and consume up to three cups per day during your menstrual cycle.

Saffron (Crocus sativus):

Saffron is a valuable herb used in various African cultures to alleviate menstrual pain. It has natural analgesic properties that can reduce both pain and discomfort. To use saffron, add a pinch of saffron threads to a cup of hot water and let it steep for 10 minutes. Drink one cup of saffron tea per day during your menstrual cycle.

African Potato (Hypoxis hemerocallidea):

Used in African traditional medicine, African potato has been reported to reduce pain associated with menstruation. The recommended dosage is generally 2-4 capsules (500mg each) per day, taken with meals. It is advisable to consult a healthcare professional before using African potato as it may interact with certain medications.

Rooibos (Aspalathus linearis):

Rooibos, a popular African herbal tea, has shown potential in alleviating menstrual pain. It has anti-inflammatory and analgesic properties that can help relax uterine muscles. To make rooibos tea, steep one tea bag or one teaspoon of dried rooibos leaves in a cup of hot water for 5-7 minutes. Consume up to three cups per day during your menstrual cycle.

Dosages mentioned above are general guidelines, and variations may occur depending on individual factors such as weight, age, and overall health. Remember to use herbal treatments as complementary options and not as a replacement for medical advice or prescribed medications.

Asian Herbal Treatments for Menstrual Pain

Rooted in traditional practices, Asian herbal treatments offer a holistic and natural approach to managing menstrual pain. In this book, we will explore some effective Asian herbal remedies, their preparations, and recommended dosages to provide women with soothing alternatives.

<u>*Dong Quai (Angelica sinensis):*</u>

- ❖ **Effectiveness**: *Dong Quai, often referred to as the "female ginseng," is a staple in traditional Chinese medicine. It is believed to regulate blood flow, alleviate menstrual cramps, and balance hormonal fluctuations.*

- ❖ **Tea**: *Brew Dong Quai tea by simmering one teaspoon of dried Dong Quai root in a cup of hot water for 15 minutes. Consume this tea once or twice a day during your menstrual cycle.*

- ❖ **Capsule and tincture**: *Dong Quai is available in both capsule and tincture forms. For capsules, a common dosage is 500-1000 mg, taken up to three times daily. Tinctures can be taken in 1-2 ml doses, mixed with water, two to three times a day.*

<u>*Turmeric (Curcuma longa):*</u>

❖ **Effectiveness**: *Turmeric contains curcumin, a compound with potent anti-inflammatory properties. This makes turmeric a valuable herb for reducing menstrual pain and inflammation.*

❖ **Tea**: *Create a turmeric tea by mixing one teaspoon of turmeric powder with hot water and honey to taste. Drink this tea once a day during menstruation for relief.*

❖ **Capsule and tincture**: *In addition to turmeric tea, turmeric supplements, typically available in capsule form, can provide a convenient and standardized dosage. A common recommendation is 500 mg to 1,000 mg of turmeric capsules two to three times a day during menstruation.*

Licorice Root (Glycyrrhiza glabra):

❖ **Effectiveness**: *Licorice root has anti-inflammatory and anti-spasmodic properties that can help alleviate menstrual cramps and discomfort.*

❖ **Preparation**: *Prepare licorice tea by steeping one teaspoon of dried licorice root in hot water for 10-15 minutes. Consume this tea once a day during your menstrual period.*

- ❖ **Tincture**: *The recommended dosage is usually 1-2 ml diluted in water, two to three times a day during the menstrual period.*

Ashwagandha (Withania somnifera):

- ❖ **Effectiveness**: *Ashwagandha is an adaptogenic herb in Ayurvedic medicine known for its ability to balance hormones and reduce stress, potentially easing menstrual pain.*
- ❖ **Powder**: *Mix one teaspoon of ashwagandha powder with warm milk and honey. Consume this mixture once daily during the week leading up to your menstrual cycle.*
- ❖ **Capsule**: *Ashwagandha is often available in capsule form. A recommended dosage is 300-500 mg of ashwagandha capsules once or twice daily, starting a week before menstruation.*

Chinese Skullcap (Scutellaria baicalensis):

- ❖ **Effectiveness**: *Chinese Skullcap is valued in traditional Chinese medicine for its anti-inflammatory properties, which may contribute to relieving menstrual cramps.*
- ❖ **Preparation**: *Create a Chinese Skullcap tea by boiling one teaspoon of dried Chinese Skullcap root in a cup of water for 10-15 minutes. Drink this tea once a day during your menstrual period.*

- ❖ **Capsules:** *Take 500 mg to 1,000 mg of Chinese skullcap capsules, depending on the product's concentration.Typically, capsules are taken two to three times a day. Start taking the capsules a few days before the expected onset of menstrual pain and continue throughout the menstrual period.*

Asian herbal treatments for menstrual pain present a rich tapestry of natural remedies that have been embraced for centuries. By incorporating these herbs into your routine and respecting individual health needs, you can tap into the wisdom of traditional Asian medicine for a more balanced and comfortable menstrual experience.

Prasaplai formula

Prasaplai formula is a traditional Thai herbal remedy that consists of a combination of ten medicinal plants and two chemical compounds. Each component contributes to the formulation, creating a complex mixture aimed at addressing menstrual pain. Let's analyze the potential effects of each ingredient:

- ❖ *Citrus hystrix DC. (Kaffir Lime Pericarp):*
  - o *May have anti-inflammatory and analgesic properties.*
- ❖ *Acorus calamus L. (Sweet Flag Root):*
  - o *Known for its anti-inflammatory and muscle-relaxant properties.*
- ❖ *Allium sativum L. (Garlic Bulb):*
  - o *Exhibits anti-inflammatory and analgesic effects.*
  - o *May have vasodilatory properties.*
- ❖ *Eleutherine americana (Aubl.) Merr. ex K. Heyne (Eleutherine Bulb):*
  - o *Traditional use for pain relief and anti-inflammatory effects.*
- ❖ *Piper nigrum L. (Black Pepper Fruit):*
  - o *Contains piperine, which may enhance the bioavailability of other compounds.*
  - o *Exhibits anti-inflammatory properties.*
- ❖ *Piper retrofractum Vahl (Long Pepper Fruit):*

- o *Known for its traditional use in pain relief and anti-inflammatory effects.*
- ❖ *Zingiber officinale Roscoe (Ginger Rhizomes):*
  - o *Well-known for its anti-inflammatory and analgesic properties.*
  - o *May help reduce menstrual pain.*
- ❖ *Curcuma zedoaria Roscoe (Zedoary Rhizomes):*
  - o *Contains curcumin, known for its anti-inflammatory effects.*
  - o *May contribute to pain relief.*
- ❖ *Nigella sativa L. (Black Seed):*
  - o *Exhibits anti-inflammatory and analgesic properties.*
- ❖ *Sodium Chloride (Salt):*
  - o *May contribute to electrolyte balance but unlikely to have a direct impact on menstrual pain.*
- ❖ *Camphor:*
  - o *Traditionally used for its analgesic and soothing effects.*
- ❖ *Zingiber cassumunar Roxb. (Cassumunar Rhizome):*
  - o *Known for its anti-inflammatory and pain-relieving properties.*

The Prasaplai formula comprises a combination of herbs with well-documented traditional uses for pain relief and anti-inflammatory effects. The inclusion of ginger, turmeric (from Zedoary rhizomes), and black pepper suggests an emphasis on targeting inflammation and pain pathways. The addition of sodium chloride and camphor may contribute to the overall formulation's properties.

It's essential to note that while these individual components have shown promising effects in preclinical studies, traditional knowledge, and anecdotal evidence, scientific research specifically on the Prasaplai formula for menstrual pain is limited. Furthermore, the effectiveness of herbal remedies can vary among individuals.

Before considering the use of the Prasaplai formula or any herbal remedy for menstrual pain, it is crucial to consult with a healthcare professional. They can provide guidance based on your medical history, potential interactions with medications, and the most current scientific evidence available.

Additionally, it's advisable to be cautious and ensure that the product is sourced from reputable manufacturers to guarantee quality and safety.

Ayurveda for Menstrual Pain

In Ayurveda, there are various herbs and formulations believed to help alleviate menstrual pain. Some common herbs include:

- ❖ **Ashoka (Saraca indica):** *Known for its uterine tonic properties, it is often used in Ayurvedic formulations for women's health.*

- ❖ **Shatavari (Asparagus racemosus):** *This herb is considered a general tonic for the female reproductive system and is often used to support hormonal balance.*

- ❖ **Lodhra (Symplocos racemosa):** *It is believed to have astringent and anti-inflammatory properties and may be used in menstrual disorders.*

- ❖ **Dashamoola:** *This is a combination of ten roots, and it is often used in Ayurveda to balance Vata and promote overall well-being.*

- ❖ **Ginger (Zingiber officinale):** *Known for its anti-inflammatory properties, ginger may help reduce pain and discomfort associated with menstruation.*

- ❖ **Turmeric (Curcuma longa):** *It has anti-inflammatory and analgesic properties and may help reduce pain.*

- ❖ **Triphala:** *A combination of three fruits (amalaki, bibhitaki, and haritaki), it is known for its detoxifying and balancing effects.*

Ayurvedic formulations are often prescribed in the form of powders, tablets, or decoctions. Dosages can vary, and it's crucial to follow the guidance of a healthcare professional. It's important to note that individual responses to herbs can vary, and the appropriate dosage may depend on various factors such as your overall health, body constitution (Prakriti), and any existing medical conditions. Dosages and specific formulations should be determined by a qualified Ayurvedic practitioner.

Kampo

Kampo is a traditional Japanese herbal medicine system that has been used for centuries. However, like Ayurveda, it's crucial to consult with a qualified healthcare professional or Kampo practitioner for personalized advice and recommendations tailored to your specific health needs. The following are some herbs commonly used in Kampo formulas for menstrual pain:

* **Tokishigyakukagoshuyushokyoto (TJ-68):** *This is a commonly prescribed Kampo formula for menstrual disorders, including pain. It contains herbs like keishibukuryogan, which is believed to have analgesic and anti-inflammatory properties.*

* **Shakuyakukanzoto (Shao Yao Gan Cao Tang):** *This formula includes peony root (shakuyaku) and licorice (kanzo), among other herbs. It is often used to address menstrual irregularities and pain.*

* **Keishibukuryogan (Gui Zhi Fu Ling Wan):** *This formula includes cinnamon twig (gui zhi) and hoelen (fu ling) and is traditionally used for gynecological issues, including menstrual pain.*

Dosages for Kampo formulas can vary based on the specific formulation, the severity of symptoms, and individual factors. Kampo formulas are often prescribed in granule or extract form, and the dosage is typically determined by a Kampo practitioner based on their assessment of your condition.

If you're interested in exploring Kampo for menstrual pain or other health concerns, consider consulting with a healthcare provider who has experience in traditional Japanese medicine or seeking out a qualified Kampo practitioner. They can provide you with personalized recommendations based on your individual health status and needs.

The Role of Enzymes in Treating Menstrual Pain

Enzymes are naturally occurring substances that play a vital role in the body's chemical processes. They act as catalysts, speeding up and facilitating numerous biochemical reactions. When it comes to treating menstrual pain, certain enzymes have shown promising effects in reducing discomfort.

One such enzyme is bromelain, which is obtained from pineapple stems.

- ❖ *Bromelain is known for its anti-inflammatory properties and has been found to effectively reduce pain associated with menstruation. It works by inhibiting the production of prostaglandins, hormone-like substances that can cause significant pain and inflammation.*

Another enzyme that has gained attention is serrapeptase, derived from the silkworm.

- ❖ *Serrapeptase has powerful anti-inflammatory effects and is commonly used to treat various types of pain, including menstrual cramps. It works by breaking down proteins that contribute to pain and inflammation, thus providing relief to women suffering from menstrual pain*

Dosage Recommendations

When using enzymes to treat menstrual pain, it is important to follow the recommended dosage guidelines. The appropriate dosage may vary depending on the specific enzyme and the severity of pain experienced.

- ❖ *For* **bromelain**, *the usual recommended dosage is around 500-1000 mg per day, taken between meals.*
- ❖ **Serrapeptase** *is typically taken in doses ranging from 10-30 mg, one to three times a day, with or without food.*

It is worth noting that while enzymes like bromelain and serrapeptase have shown promise in relieving menstrual pain, their effectiveness may vary from person to person. Some women may experience significant relief, while others may find minimal benefits. It is always advisable to consult with a healthcare professional who can provide personalized advice based on your specific circumstances.

Considerations and Precaution

While enzymes can be a safe and effective option for treating menstrual pain, it is essential to consider certain precautions and potential side effects. Individuals with allergies to certain foods, especially pineapple or silk, should exercise caution when using bromelain or serrapeptase. Allergic reactions may range from mild to severe and can include symptoms such as itching, rash, or difficulty breathing. If any adverse effects are experienced, it is recommended to discontinue use and seek medical advice.

Amino Acids: An Effective Treatment for Menstrual Pain

Amino acids are the building blocks of proteins, essential for various physiological processes in the body. Studies have shown that certain amino acids play a crucial role in reducing inflammation and muscle spasms, making them effective in alleviating menstrual pain. Their mechanisms of action, such as reducing inflammation, improving blood circulation, and relieving muscle spasms, make them effective alternatives to traditional pain relievers.

- ❖ **L-arginine:** One such amino acid is L-arginine, which acts as a vasodilator by increasing the production of nitric oxide. This dilation of blood vessels helps to improve blood flow to the uterus and reduce the intensity of menstrual cramps.

- ❖ **L-taurine:** Another amino acid, L-taurine, exhibits anti-inflammatory properties. It helps to reduce the production of prostaglandins, which are hormone-like substances responsible for triggering uterine contractions leading to menstrual pain.

- ❖ **L-carnitine,** an amino acid derivative, has been shown to enhance blood circulation, reduce pain intensity, and improve mood during menstruation. It works by *increasing energy production within the cells, thereby reducing muscle fatigue and discomfort.*

Dosage Recommendations

When it comes to using amino acids for menstrual pain relief, it is essential to consult with a healthcare professional or a qualified practitioner to determine the appropriate dosage. The dosage can vary depending on individual factors such as age, weight, and overall health.

- *In general, the recommended dosage for* **L-arginine** *is around 4-6 grams per day. It is commonly available in supplement form and can be taken throughout the menstrual cycle, starting a few days before the expected onset of pain.*
- **L-taurine** *is typically recommended at a dosage of 500-2000 mg per day. It can be consumed as a stand-alone supplement or found in combination with other amino acids in menstrual support formulations.*
- **L-carnitine** *is often suggested at a dosage of 500-1000 mg per day, starting a few days before menstruation begins and continuing throughout the cycle.*

By considering an individual's unique needs and following the recommended dosages, amino acids can provide relief and contribute to a better quality of life during menstruation.

Herbal Oil Massage: A Natural Approach to Alleviating Menstrual Pain

Herbal oil massage has been used for centuries in various traditional healing systems to soothe aching muscles and reduce pain. When it comes to menstrual pain, a carefully chosen blend of herbal oils can provide several benefits:

- ✓ **Muscle Relaxation:** *The gentle and soothing massage movements, combined with the properties of herbal oils, help relax the muscles of the lower abdomen and lower back, reducing cramping and discomfort.*

- ✓ **Improved Blood Circulation:** *The massaging action stimulates blood flow to the pelvic region, improving oxygenation and nutrient supply to the uterus and surrounding tissues. This increased circulation can relieve congestion and reduce pain.*

- ✓ **Hormonal Balance:** *Certain herbs used in the oils, such as clary sage and lavender, are believed to have hormone-regulating properties. These herbs can help balance hormonal fluctuations during the menstrual cycle and mitigate symptoms such as mood swings and irritability.*

Preparations and Application

To prepare herbal oil for menstrual pain relief, you will need a carrier oil such as sesame, coconut, or almond oil and a selection of pain-reducing herbs. Some commonly used herbs for menstrual pain include:

- ❖ **Clary Sage***: Known for its soothing properties, clary sage helps relax muscles and balance hormones.*
- ❖ **Lavender***: Renowned for its calming effects, lavender oil can help reduce stress and promote relaxation.*
- ❖ **Marjoram***: This herb has analgesic properties and can be beneficial in reducing pain and supporting muscle relaxation.*
- ❖ **Chamomile** *oil is derived from the flowers of the chamomile plant (Matricaria chamomilla). It is popular for its soothing and anti-inflammatory properties and can be used topically to relieve menstrual pain.*

To make the herbal oil, follow these steps:

- ○ *Choose a clean and dry glass jar with an airtight lid.*
- ○ *Fill the jar halfway with your chosen carrier oil.*
- ○ *Add a few drops of each herbal oil, such as clary sage, lavender, and marjoram. The exact number of drops may vary depending on personal preference and the potency of the oils.*

o   *Close the jar tightly and shake well to combine the oils.*

o   *Let the mixture sit for a few days to allow the oils to infuse.*

<u>*To apply the herbal oil:*</u>

- o *Warm the oil slightly by placing the jar in a bowl of warm water. Be cautious not to heat it too much to avoid burns.*
- o *Lie down in a comfortable position and apply the warmed oil to the lower abdomen and lower back.*
- o *Gently massage the area in circular motions, using light to moderate pressure.*
- o *Continue the massage for about 10-15 minutes, focusing on the areas where the pain is most intense.*
- o *After the massage, you can rest for a while to allow the oil to penetrate the skin and provide maximum benefits.*

Dosage Recommendations

There is no specific dosage recommendation for herbal oil massage, as it varies from person to person. It is recommended to perform the massage once or twice a day, starting a few days before the expected onset of menstrual pain, and continuing throughout the menstrual cycle.

Remember that everyone's body is unique, and it is essential to listen to your own comfort levels. If any irritation or adverse reactions occur, discontinue use and consult a healthcare professional.

Bowen Technique for the Treatment of Menstrual Pain: Mechanism of Action and Dosage

The Bowen Technique is a complementary therapy that involves gentle and non-invasive moves over precise points or areas of the body. The technique works by stimulating the nervous system to reset and balance itself, reducing tension and increasing vitality. Bowen moves mobilize the fascia, a thin sheath covering the muscles and organs, thereby facilitating the movement of lymph and blood, and improving the body's natural healing ability.

*During a **Bowen session**, the practitioner uses thumb and fingers to apply gentle rolling and stretching movements to specific areas, focusing on the lower back, pelvis, and upper legs. These areas contain nerve endings that connect with the reproductive system, including the ovaries, uterus, and fallopian tubes. Bowen moves aim to reset the autonomic nervous system, reduce muscular tension and spasm, and improve circulation to the pelvic and reproductive organs, thereby relieving menstrual pain.*

Dosage

The Bowen Technique is individualized to suit each patient's unique needs. The practitioner usually recommends a course of four to six weekly sessions, followed by additional sessions as needed. Each session lasts approximately 30 to 45 minutes, with the patient lying down and dressed in light, non-restrictive clothing.

Effectiveness

Although limited research studies have been conducted on the effectiveness of Bowen Technique for menstrual pain, anecdotal evidence suggests that the technique may provide relief from menstrual cramps, back pain, and other related symptoms. The Bowen Technique is considered safe and gentle and may be used alone or in combination with other therapies. The Bowen Technique is a complementary therapy that may be useful in treating menstrual pain. The technique involves gentle and non-invasive moves that stimulate the nervous system and facilitate the movement of lymph and blood, thereby reducing tension and increasing vitality. The Bowen Technique is individualized for each patient, and a course of four to six weekly sessions is usually recommended.

Vitamins and minerals

Addressing hormonal imbalances that contribute to menstrual pain can involve a combination of herbs, supplements, and lifestyle modifications. It's important to note that individual responses to these treatments can vary, and consulting with a healthcare professional is advisable, especially if you have pre-existing medical conditions or are taking medications. Here are some natural approaches to address hormonal imbalances and alleviate menstrual pain:

<u>*Omega-3 Fatty Acids:*</u>
- ❖ **Mechanism**: *Omega-3 fatty acids, found in fish oil and flaxseed oil, have anti-inflammatory properties that may help reduce the production of inflammatory prostaglandins, easing menstrual pain.*
- ❖ **Dosage**: *Consider incorporating omega-3 supplements into your diet. A typical dosage might be 1,000-2,000 mg of EPA and DHA combined per day.*

<u>*Magnesium:*</u>
- ❖ **Mechanism**: *Magnesium helps regulate muscle function and may alleviate cramping by relaxing the smooth muscles of the uterus.*

❖ **Dosage**: *Take magnesium supplements, such as magnesium citrate or magnesium glycinate. A common dosage is around 200-400 mg per day. Start with a lower dose and gradually increase to avoid digestive issues.*

<u>**B-vitamins:**</u>

❖ **Mechanism**: *B-vitamins, especially B6 (pyridoxine), are involved in hormonal balance. They may help alleviate premenstrual symptoms, including pain.*

❖ **Dosage**: *B-complex supplements containing a range of B-vitamins, including B6, can be beneficial. The recommended dosage varies, but a common dose is around 50 mg of B6 per day.*

Illuminating Relief: Exploring Light Therapy and Wavelengths for Easing Menstrual Pain

Menstrual pain, a common concern for many women, often prompts a search for effective and non-invasive therapies. One emerging area of interest is light therapy, which utilizes specific wavelengths of light to address various health issues. In this book, we will delve into the different types of light therapy and the wavelengths applied for treating menstrual pain.

Types of Light Therapy:

- ❖ **Red Light Therapy:**
  - ○ *Red light therapy, also known as low-level laser therapy (LLLT) or photobiomodulation, utilizes red or near-infrared light to penetrate tissues and stimulate cellular activity.*
  - ○ *Wavelengths in the range of 620 to 700 nm are commonly used in red light therapy. This range has shown anti-inflammatory effects*

and may aid in reducing pain associated with menstrual cramps.

- ❖ **Blue Light Therapy:**
  - ○ *Blue light therapy is often used to treat conditions such as acne and seasonal affective disorder (SAD). It works by targeting specific molecules in the skin and has potential applications in pain management.*
  - ○ *While the primary focus of blue light therapy is not menstrual pain, some studies suggest that its anti-inflammatory properties might contribute to pain reduction.*
- ❖ **Infrared Light Therapy:**
  - ○ *Infrared light therapy involves the use of longer wavelengths than red light therapy, typically ranging from 700 nm to 1 mm.*
  - ○ *Infrared light penetrates deeper into tissues and may enhance blood circulation, potentially addressing the ischemic component of menstrual pain.*
- ❖ **Full-Spectrum Light:**
  - ○ *Full-spectrum light includes all colors in the visible light spectrum, mimicking natural sunlight. Exposure to full-spectrum light is commonly used to address conditions like seasonal depression.*

o *The potential impact of full-spectrum light on mood and hormonal balance may indirectly contribute to managing menstrual pain.*

Scientific Basis:

The application of light therapy for menstrual pain is grounded in the understanding of how light interacts with cells and tissues. Studies suggest that specific wavelengths of light can modulate cellular functions, influencing factors such as inflammation, blood flow, and the release of neurotransmitters.

Practical Applications:

- ❖ **Natural Sunlight Exposure:** *Spending time outdoors in natural sunlight, especially during the morning, can positively influence circadian rhythms and provide exposure to beneficial light wavelengths.*

- ❖ **Light Boxes:** *Light boxes, often used for conditions like SAD, emit bright light and may be beneficial for individuals with menstrual pain. These devices are designed to mimic natural sunlight and are used for short daily sessions.*

- ❖ **Wearable Light Devices:** *Advancements in technology have led to the development of wearable light devices that can be worn as accessories. These devices emit specific wavelengths of light and can be incorporated into daily routines.*

- ❖ **Clinical Light Therapy Sessions:** *Some healthcare facilities offer light therapy as part of pain* *management protocols. Clinically administered light therapy sessions, especially those involving targeted wavelengths, may provide more controlled and potent relief.*

* ❖ **Combination Therapies:** *Combining light therapy with other non-invasive treatments, such as heat therapy or relaxation techniques, may enhance the overall effectiveness of menstrual pain management.*

Before embarking on light therapy for menstrual pain, individuals should consult with healthcare professionals, including gynecologists and pain specialists. They can provide guidance on the appropriateness of light therapy based on an individual's health history and the severity of menstrual pain. Light therapy, with its diverse applications and potential benefits, represents a promising avenue for managing menstrual pain.

Oxygen

While it is true that oxygen plays a crucial role in various physiological processes, and there is evidence supporting the use of oxygen therapy for certain medical conditions, the application of oxygen specifically for alleviating menstrual cramps is not a well-established or widely recognized practice within the medical community.

Menstrual cramps, also known as dysmenorrhea, are primarily caused by the release of prostaglandins, hormone-like substances that prompt the uterus to contract. The pain associated with menstrual cramps is largely attributed to these contractions and the resultant reduction in blood flow, leading to temporary oxygen deprivation in the uterine muscles.

The concept that increased oxygen delivery to the uterus could potentially alleviate menstrual cramps by addressing oxygen deprivation is intriguing. However, the practicality and effectiveness of delivering oxygen to the uterus in a targeted and controlled manner, such as through external oxygen therapy, present challenges.

However there are some anegdotal evidence that OTC oxygen helped to alleviate pain, either due oxygen supply or placebo.

Homeopathy

Homeopathy is a system of alternative medicine that utilizes highly diluted substances derived from plants, minerals, or animals to stimulate the body's self-healing abilities. In the context of menstrual pain, various homeopathic remedies are commonly recommended. It is crucial to consult with a qualified homeopath or healthcare professional for personalized advice and accurate dosage recommendations. The following is an overview of some commonly used homeopathic preparations for menstrual pain.

Common Homeopathic Remedies for Menstrual Pain:

- ❖ **Pulsatilla (Wind Flower):**
    - ○ *Symptoms:* **Changeable moods, weepiness, and a desire for open air.**
    - ○ *Dosage:* **Typically available in various potencies (6C, 30C, etc.). A common recommendation might be 3 pellets of 30C every 2-4 hours during the pain.**
- ❖ **Sepia (Cuttlefish Ink):**
    - ○ *Symptoms:* **Irritability, fatigue, and a feeling of heaviness in the pelvic area.**
    - ○ *Dosage:* **Similar to Pulsatilla, it is available in different potencies. A standard dose may be 3 pellets of 30C every 4-6 hours.**

- ❖ **Mag Phos (Magnesium Phosphate):**
  - o *Symptoms:* **Cramping pains that are relieved by warmth and pressure.**
  - o *Dosage:* **Often recommended in a low potency such as 6X or 6C. A typical suggestion might be 3-5 pellets every 15 minutes during acute pain.**
- ❖ **Caulophyllum (Blue Cohosh):**
  - o *Symptoms:* **Severe cramps, irregular menstruation.**
  - o *Dosage:* **Usually in low potencies like 6C or 12C. A common recommendation might be 3 pellets every 1-2 hours during pain.**
- ❖ **Belladonna (Deadly Nightshade):**
  - o *Symptoms:* **Sudden, intense pain with heat and throbbing.**
  - o *Dosage:* **Typically available in various potencies. A standard recommendation might be 3 pellets of 30C every 2-3 hours during intense pain.**

Dosage Guidelines:

Potency: *Homeopathic remedies come in various potencies, such as 6C, 30C, 200C, etc. The choice of potency depends on the individual's symptoms and the severity of the condition. Lower potencies (6C-30C) are often used for acute conditions, while higher potencies (200C and above) may be prescribed for chronic issues.*

Frequency: *The frequency of dosage depends on the intensity of symptoms. During acute pain, it's common to take the remedy every 15-60 minutes initially and then space out as symptoms improve. For chronic conditions, a lower frequency such as 1-3 times a day might be appropriate.*

Administration: *Homeopathic remedies are typically in the form of small pellets. It's recommended to let them dissolve under the tongue. Avoid handling the pellets to prevent contamination.*

Important Considerations:

Individualization: *Homeopathy emphasizes treating the individual, not the disease. The choice of remedy is based on the person's unique symptoms, mental and emotional state, and overall constitution.*

Consult a Professional: *While homeopathic remedies are generally considered safe, it's crucial to consult with a qualified homeopath or healthcare professional. They can provide a thorough evaluation and recommend the most suitable remedy and dosage for your specific case.*

Adjunct to Conventional Care: *Homeopathic remedies can be used as complementary therapy alongside conventional medical treatments. Always inform your healthcare providers about any complementary therapies you are using.*

In conclusion, homeopathy offers a holistic approach to menstrual pain, considering not just the physical symptoms but also the emotional and mental aspects of the individual. The effectiveness of homeopathic remedies can vary from person to person, and consulting with a qualified homeopath ensures a tailored and safe approach to managing menstrual discomfort.

Yoga for Menstrual Pain: Harnessing the Healing Power of Asanas

Menstrual pain, also known as dysmenorrhea, is a common concern for many women. While there are various approaches to managing this discomfort, yoga offers a holistic and natural way to alleviate menstrual cramps and promote overall well-being. In this book, we'll explore the benefits of yoga for menstrual pain and recommend specific asanas (yoga poses) that may help ease discomfort.

The Benefits of Yoga for Menstrual Pain:

- ✓ **Relief from Muscle Tension:** *Menstrual cramps often result from the contraction of uterine muscles. Yoga poses help release tension in the pelvic area and promote relaxation, reducing the intensity of cramps.*

- ✓ **Improved Blood Circulation:** *Many yoga poses enhance blood circulation, which can alleviate congestion in the pelvic region and minimize the severity of menstrual pain.*

- ✓ **Hormonal Balance:** *Yoga is known to have a positive impact on hormonal balance. Certain poses stimulate the endocrine system, potentially helping to regulate* *hormonal fluctuations associated with the menstrual cycle.*

✓ **Stress Reduction:** *Stress can exacerbate menstrual pain. Yoga practices, including breathwork and meditation, help activate the parasympathetic nervous system, promoting relaxation and stress reduction.*

✓ **Increased Mind-Body Awareness:** *Yoga encourages mindfulness and a deeper connection between the mind and body. This heightened awareness may help women better understand and manage their menstrual symptoms.*

Recommended Yoga Asanas for Menstrual Pain:

❖ **Child's Pose (Balasana):**
  - ○ *How to do it: Kneel on the mat, sit back on your heels, and then slowly fold forward, reaching your arms in front of you. Rest your forehead on the mat.*
  - ○ *Benefits: Stretches the lower back, hips, and thighs, promoting relaxation and relieving tension.*

❖ **Cat-Cow Stretch (Marjarasana):**
  - ○ *How to do it: Start on your hands and knees. Inhale as you arch your back (cow pose), and exhale as you round your spine (cat pose).*

- o *Benefits: Enhances flexibility in the spine, alleviates back discomfort, and massages the abdominal organs.*

❖ **Supine Bound Angle Pose (Supta Baddha Konasana):**
  - o *How to do it: Lie on your back, bend your knees, and bring the soles of your feet together. Allow your knees to fall outward.*
  - o *Benefits: Opens the hips and groins, promoting relaxation and reducing tension in the pelvic area.*

❖ **Bridge Pose (Setu Bandhasana):**
  - o *How to do it: Lie on your back, bend your knees, and lift your hips towards the ceiling.*
  - o *Benefits: Strengthens the pelvic muscles, improves circulation, and relieves backache.*

❖ **Legs Up the Wall Pose (Viparita Karani):**
  - o *How to do it: Sit sideways against a wall, then swing your legs up so that your back is on the floor and your legs are resting against the wall.*
  - o *Benefits: Facilitates blood circulation, reduces menstrual cramps, and promotes relaxation.*

❖ **Reclining Bound Angle Pose (Supta Baddha Konasana):**
  - o *How to do it: Lie on your back, bring the soles of your feet together, and let your knees fall outward.*

o   *Benefits: Stretches the inner thighs and groins, releases tension in the hips, and provides relief from menstrual discomfort.*

Tips for Practicing Yoga During Menstruation:

- o   **Listen to Your Body:** *Pay attention to how your body feels, and modify or skip poses that cause discomfort.*
- o   **Gentle Movement:** *Opt for gentle and restorative yoga practices during the menstrual period to support the body's natural healing process.*
- o   **Use Props:** *Props such as bolsters and blankets can enhance comfort and relaxation during yoga poses.*

Conclusion:

Yoga provides a holistic and gentle approach to managing menstrual pain, addressing both the physical and emotional aspects of discomfort. The recommended asanas, when practiced mindfully, can contribute to relieving tension, improving circulation, and fostering a sense of well-being during the menstrual cycle. As with any exercise regimen, it's advisable to consult with a healthcare professional before beginning a new yoga practice, especially if you have underlying health conditions. Remember that individual experiences may vary, and finding what works best for your body is key to incorporating yoga into your menstrual wellness routine.

Finding Balance and Relief: The Power of Tai Chi for Menstrual Pain

Tai Chi, also known as Tai Chi Chuan, is an ancient Chinese martial art that combines slow, graceful movements with focused breathing and meditation. This centuries-old practice has been hailed for its ability to foster physical, mental, and emotional well-being. When applied to menstrual pain treatment, Tai Chi offers a gentle yet powerful approach that can help restore balance to your body and alleviate discomfort.

How Tai Chi Works for Menstrual Pain Relief

- ✓ **Enhancing Circulation:** *Tai Chi's flowing, rhythmic movements stimulate blood circulation throughout the body, including the reproductive system. Improved circulation can help reduce the intensity of menstrual cramps and alleviate pain.*

- ✓ **Stress Reduction:** *Stress can exacerbate menstrual pain by tightening muscles and increasing inflammation. Tai Chi, with its emphasis on deep breathing and relaxation, helps to reduce stress levels. As you flow through the gentle movements, you enter a state of* *calm, activating the body's natural healing response and easing menstrual pain.*

- ✓ **Muscle Relaxation:** *Tai Chi promotes gentle stretching and postural alignment, helping to release tension and loosen tight muscles. By targeting the lower back, abdomen, and pelvic area, Tai Chi can alleviate cramps and contribute to overall pain reduction.*

- ✓ **Balancing Hormones:** *Regular practice of Tai Chi has been shown to support hormone balance, an essential factor for regulating the menstrual cycle. By harnessing the mind-body connection, Tai Chi aids in harmonizing hormone production, reducing the severity of menstrual symptoms.*

- ✓ **Improving Overall Well-being:** *Beyond pain relief, Tai Chi offers a myriad of additional benefits. It boosts energy levels, improves mental focus, cultivates mindfulness, and enhances body awareness. These positive effects can contribute to a more positive outlook during menstruation, easing emotional fluctuations and promoting a sense of overall well-being.*

Getting Started with Tai Chi for Menstrual Pain Relief

To begin your Tai Chi journey for menstrual pain relief, consider the following steps:

- o **Find a Qualified Instructor:** *Look for a qualified Tai Chi instructor who has experience in working with women's health or menstrual issues. They can guide you in learning the proper postures, movements, and breathing techniques specific to alleviating menstrual pain.*

- o **Practice Regularly:** *Consistency is key. Aim for regular Tai Chi practice, ideally a few times a week, to experience the cumulative benefits. Start with shorter sessions and gradually increase the duration as you become more comfortable.*

- o **Combine with Other Holistic Approaches:** *Tai Chi can be complemented by other natural remedies such as herbal teas, heat therapy, acupuncture, and dietary adjustments. Consult with a healthcare professional or holistic practitioner for a personalized approach to managing your menstrual pain.*

- o **Listen to Your Body:** *Adapt your Tai Chi practice to suit your individual needs on any given day. Modify movements or take breaks as necessary. Remember, Tai Chi is about fluidity and finding your own balance.*

Conclusion

Tai Chi offers a gentle, holistic approach to menstrual pain treatment, providing relief while nurturing your entire body and mind. This ancient practice empowers women to reclaim control over their menstrual cycles, restoring balance, and promoting overall well-being. By embracing Tai Chi, you can tap into the power of movement, breath, and mindfulness to find harmony within, easing the discomforts of menstruation and enhancing your quality of life. Embark on this transformative journey and discover the profound healing potential of Tai Chi for menstrual pain relief.

Acupuncture for Menstrual Pain: A Traditional Healing Approach for Prevention and Immediate Relief

Acupuncture is a traditional Chinese medicine practice that involves inserting thin needles into specific points on the body to stimulate energy flow, or Qi. According to traditional Chinese medicine, the smooth flow of Qi is vital for maintaining balance and good health. When there is a blockage or imbalance in the flow of Qi, it can result in various health issues, including menstrual pain.

Prevention Through Regular Sessions:

- ✓ **Balancing Qi and Blood Flow:** *Acupuncture aims to balance the flow of Qi and blood in the body. By addressing any imbalances before the onset of menstruation, regular acupuncture sessions can potentially reduce the severity of menstrual cramps.*

- ✓ **Regulating Hormones:** *Acupuncture has been shown to influence the endocrine system, including hormones associated with the menstrual cycle. This regulation can contribute to a more harmonious menstrual cycle and alleviate symptoms like cramping.*

✓ **Stress Reduction:** *Acupuncture is known for its ability to promote relaxation and reduce stress. Chronic stress can exacerbate menstrual pain, so incorporating acupuncture into your routine can provide both mental and physical relief.*

Acupuncture for Immediate Relief:

❖ **Lower Abdominal Points:** *Acupuncture points in the lower abdomen can directly address menstrual pain. Needles may be strategically placed to alleviate muscle tension and reduce cramping sensations.*

❖ **Spleen 6 (SP6):** *Located on the inner side of the lower leg, about three finger-widths above the ankle bone, SP6 is believed to regulate the menstrual cycle, alleviate pain, and address conditions related to the reproductive system.*

❖ **Liver 3 (LV3):** *Found on the top of the foot between the big toe and the second toe, LV3 is thought to promote the smooth flow of Qi and blood, addressing menstrual pain and emotional imbalances.*

❖ **Governing Vessel 4 (GV4):** *Situated on the lower abdomen, GV4 is associated with the reproductive organs. Stimulation of this point may help regulate menstrual flow and reduce pain.*

❖ **Conception Vessel 6 (CV6):** *Located two finger-widths below the navel, CV6 is believed to tonify the reproductive system and relieve abdominal discomfort.*

Acupuncture offers a time-tested and holistic approach to managing menstrual pain, providing both prevention through regular sessions and immediate relief during menstruation. By promoting the balance of Qi, regulating hormones, and reducing stress, acupuncture addresses the root causes of menstrual discomfort. As with any alternative therapy, it's essential to consult with a qualified and experienced acupuncturist, especially if you have underlying health conditions or concerns. Embrace the ancient wisdom of acupuncture to empower yourself with a natural and effective solution for navigating the challenges of menstrual pain.

Harnessing the Power of Heat: Effective Strategies for Treating Menstrual Pain

Heat therapy, or thermotherapy, involves the application of heat to soothe and relax muscles, reduce pain, and improve blood circulation. When it comes to menstrual pain, the warmth helps to ease muscle cramps and tension in the pelvic area, providing a comforting and effective form of relief.

How Heat Works for Menstrual Pain:

- ✓ **Muscle Relaxation:** *Heat promotes the relaxation of muscles, which can be particularly beneficial for alleviating the uterine contractions responsible for menstrual cramps. Relaxed muscles contribute to a reduction in pain and discomfort.*

- ✓ **Improved Blood Circulation:** *Heat helps to dilate blood vessels, improving blood flow to the affected area. Increased circulation can enhance the delivery of oxygen and nutrients to the pelvic region, aiding in the natural healing process.*

- ✓ **Reduced Nerve Sensitivity:** *Heat can decrease the sensitivity of pain receptors, providing relief from the heightened sensation of menstrual pain. This reduction* *in nerve sensitivity contributes to an overall sense of comfort.*

Methods of Applying Heat:

- ❖ **Hot Water Bottle or Heating Pad:**
    - ○ *Fill a hot water bottle with warm (not boiling) water or use an electric heating pad.*
    - ○ *Place the hot water bottle or heating pad on your lower abdomen for 15-20 minutes.*
    - ○ *Repeat as needed throughout the day.*
- ❖ **Warm Bath:**
    - ○ *Fill a bathtub with warm water.*
    - ○ *Soak in the warm bath for 15-20 minutes, allowing the heat to penetrate and relax your muscles.*
    - ○ *Add calming elements like Epsom salts or essential oils for an extra soothing experience.*
- ❖ **Heat Wraps or Patches:**
    - ○ *Disposable heat wraps or patches designed for menstrual pain relief can be applied directly to your lower abdomen.*
    - ○ *These are convenient for on-the-go relief and can provide continuous warmth for several hours.*
- ❖ **Warm Compress:**

o *Soak a clean cloth in warm water, wring out excess water, and place it on your lower abdomen.*

o *Cover the warm compress with a dry towel to retain the heat.*

o *Reheat the cloth as needed.*

❖ **DIY Rice Sock:**

o *Fill a clean sock with uncooked rice.*

o *Microwave the sock for 1-2 minutes until it reaches a comfortably warm temperature.*

o *Place the rice sock on your lower abdomen for relief.*

Heat therapy stands as a simple yet powerful method for relieving menstrual pain without resorting to medications. Whether using a hot water bottle, taking a warm bath, or applying heat patches, integrating heat therapy into your menstrual care routine can significantly improve your comfort during menstruation. As with any form of self-care, it's essential to listen to your body and choose the method that works best for you. Embrace the warmth, relax, and let the soothing power of heat guide you through your menstrual cycle with greater ease.

Empowering Wellness: Exercise and Stretching for Treating Menstrual Pain

Menstrual pain, also known as dysmenorrhea, is a common phenomenon experienced by many women during their menstrual cycle. While reaching for painkillers is a common response, incorporating exercise and stretching into your routine can offer a natural and holistic approach to managing menstrual discomfort. In this in-depth book, we will explore the benefits of exercise and stretching, specific techniques that can alleviate menstrual pain, and the science behind their effectiveness.

Benefits of Exercise for Menstrual Pain:

- ✓ **Endorphin Release:** *Exercise stimulates the release of endorphins, which act as natural pain relievers. The "feel-good" chemicals produced during physical activity can counteract the discomfort associated with menstrual cramps.*

- ✓ **Improved Blood Circulation:** *Engaging in cardiovascular exercises such as walking, jogging, or cycling enhances blood circulation. Improved* *circulation ensures that oxygen and nutrients reach the pelvic area, reducing muscle tension and cramping.*

✓ **Reduced Stress Levels:** *Stress exacerbates menstrual pain. Exercise, particularly activities like yoga or tai chi, promotes relaxation and reduces stress, contributing to overall well-being.*

✓ **Enhanced Mood and Energy Levels:** *Menstrual pain can be accompanied by mood swings and fatigue. Regular exercise has been linked to improved mood and increased energy levels, counteracting these common menstrual symptoms.*

Stretching Techniques for Menstrual Pain Relief:

- ❖ **Pelvic Tilts:**
    - ○ *Lie on your back with knees bent.*
    - ○ *Tighten your abdominal muscles and push your lower back into the floor.*
    - ○ *Hold for a few seconds and release.*
    - ○ *Repeat 10-15 times.*
- ❖ **Cat-Cow Stretch:**
    - ○ *Start on your hands and knees.*
    - ○ *Arch your back up (like a cat) and then lower it down, lifting your head and tailbone (like a cow).*
    - ○ *Repeat in a flowing motion for 5-10 minutes.*
- ❖ **Child's Pose:**

- o   *Kneel on the floor, sit back on your heels, and stretch your arms forward.*
  - o   *Lower your chest toward the floor, reaching your arms as far as comfortable.*
  - o   *Hold for 30 seconds to 1 minute.*
- ❖ **Seated Forward Bend:**
  - o   *Sit with your legs extended in front of you.*
  - o   *Hinge at your hips and reach forward towards your toes.*
  - o   *Hold for 30 seconds, breathing deeply.*
- ❖ **Butterfly Stretch:**
  - o   *Sit with your knees bent and feet together.*
  - o   *Hold your feet and gently press your knees towards the floor.*
  - o   *Hold for 1-2 minutes.*

Exercise and stretching emerge as powerful tools in the natural management of menstrual pain. By promoting endorphin release, improving blood circulation, reducing stress, and addressing muscle tension, these activities offer holistic relief. It's crucial to listen to your body, choosing activities that align with your comfort level. Integrating regular exercise and stretching into your routine can empower you to navigate your menstrual cycle with greater ease, promoting not only physical well-being but also emotional and mental balance. Embrace the transformative potential of movement and stretching to cultivate a healthier, more comfortable menstrual experience.

Healing Hands: Massage and Chiropractic Techniques for Easing Menstrual Pain

Among the diverse array of options, massage and chiropractic techniques stand out as therapeutic interventions that focus on the body's structural and muscular aspects. In this book, we will explore various massage and chiropractic techniques, how they work, and their potential benefits in easing menstrual pain.

How Massage and Chiropractic Techniques Help:

- ✓ **Increased Blood Flow:** *Both massage and chiropractic care can enhance blood circulation to the pelvic region, reducing muscle tension and promoting relaxation. Improved blood flow may contribute to a decrease in the intensity of menstrual cramps.*

- ✓ **Muscle Relaxation:** *Massage techniques, particularly those focused on the abdomen and lower back, can induce muscle relaxation. This is beneficial for alleviating the muscular tightness and spasms associated with menstrual pain.*

✓ **Nervous System Modulation:** *Chiropractic adjustments influence the nervous system, potentially modulating pain signals and reducing the perception of menstrual pain. This is achieved by addressing spinal misalignments that may impact nerve function.*

✓ **Holistic Approach:** *Both massage and chiropractic care adopt a holistic approach to health, considering the interconnectedness of the musculoskeletal system and overall well-being. This comprehensive perspective can contribute to more effective and lasting relief.*

Massage Techniques:

❖ **Abdominal Massage:**

- o *Involves gentle, circular motions applied to the lower abdomen. This technique aims to increase blood flow to the pelvic region, easing muscle tension and reducing cramping.*
- o *Therapists may use aromatherapy oils, such as lavender or chamomile, known for their relaxation properties during abdominal massage.*

❖ **Swedish Massage:**

- o *Employs long, gliding strokes, kneading, and circular motions to promote relaxation and improve blood circulation.*

- o *When applied to the lower back and pelvic area, it may help alleviate tension and reduce the intensity of menstrual cramps.*
- ❖ **Trigger Point Therapy:**
  - o *Trigger points are specific areas of muscle tightness that can refer pain to other parts of the body. Therapists use pressure and release techniques to deactivate these trigger points, potentially relieving referred pain associated with menstrual cramps.*
- ❖ **Lymphatic Drainage Massage:**
  - o *Focuses on promoting the flow of lymph, a fluid that carries waste products away from tissues. This technique can reduce fluid retention and bloating associated with menstrual cycles.*

Chiropractic Techniques:

- ❖ **Spinal Adjustments:**
  - o *Chiropractors perform spinal adjustments to correct misalignments (subluxations) in the spine. Misalignments can affect nerve function and may contribute to pelvic pain and discomfort.*
  - o *Adjustments in the lumbar and sacral regions can potentially relieve tension in the pelvic area, reducing menstrual pain.*

- ❖ Pelvic Adjustments:
  - o *Chiropractors may employ specific techniques to adjust the pelvic region directly. This can help address musculoskeletal imbalances and reduce pressure on the reproductive organs, potentially providing relief from menstrual discomfort.*
- ❖ Soft Tissue Therapy:
  - o *Soft tissue therapies, including myofascial release and massage techniques, are often incorporated into chiropractic care. These methods focus on releasing tension in muscles and connective tissues, contributing to overall pain reduction.*
- ❖ Nutritional Counseling:
  - o *Chiropractors may provide nutritional guidance to address inflammation and hormonal imbalances that contribute to menstrual pain. Dietary changes and supplements may be recommended to support overall well-being.*

Consultation with Healthcare Professionals: *Before seeking massage or chiropractic care for menstrual pain, it's crucial to consult with healthcare professionals, especially if there are underlying medical conditions.*

Individualized Treatment Plans: *Massage and chiropractic care should be tailored to individual needs. A thorough assessment by qualified practitioners ensures that treatment plans are personalized for maximum effectiveness.*
Regular Maintenance: *Regular sessions may be necessary to maintain the benefits of massage and chiropractic care for menstrual pain. Consistency in treatment can contribute to long-term relief.*

Massage and chiropractic techniques offer valuable, non-invasive approaches to managing menstrual pain. By addressing muscle tension, promoting blood flow, and modulating the nervous system, these hands-on therapies contribute to a holistic and natural approach to menstrual health. As with any alternative therapy, it is essential to consult with healthcare professionals to ensure that these techniques are appropriate for individual needs. With the healing touch of massage and chiropractic care, individuals can embrace a path to menstrual pain relief that prioritizes the body's innate capacity for balance and well-being.

Exploring TENS Devices: A Comprehensive Guide to Treating Menstrual Pain

TENS therapy involves the use of a small, battery-powered device that delivers low-voltage electrical currents through electrodes placed on the skin. These electrical impulses work to disrupt pain signals and stimulate the production of endorphins, the body's natural painkillers.

Different Types of TENS Devices:

- ❖ **Traditional TENS Devices:**
  - o *These are the most common TENS devices and are available over-the-counter for home use.*
  - o *Traditional TENS units typically have adjustable settings for intensity, frequency, and duration.*
  - o *Electrodes are placed on or near the area of pain, creating a targeted approach.*
- ❖ **Wearable TENS Devices:**
  - o *These devices are compact and designed to be worn discreetly, offering portability and convenience.*
  - o *Some wearable TENS devices are wireless, providing freedom of movement during use.*

- *They are often controlled through smartphone apps, allowing users to customize settings.*

❖ **Menstrual Pain-Specific TENS Devices:**
- *Some TENS devices are specifically designed for menstrual pain relief.*
- *These devices may come with pre-set programs or settings tailored to address the unique characteristics of menstrual cramps.*
- *They often include features like heat therapy or vibration for added comfort.*

❖ **Dual Channel TENS Devices:**
- *Dual channel TENS units have two sets of electrodes, allowing users to target multiple areas simultaneously.*
- *This type of device is beneficial for individuals experiencing widespread pain during menstruation.*

How TENS Devices Work for Menstrual Pain:

✓ **Pain Signal Disruption:**
- *TENS units work by sending electrical impulses through the skin to disrupt pain signals traveling along nerve pathways.*
- *The stimulation of nerves can lead to a reduction in the perception of pain, providing relief during menstrual cramps.*

✓ **Endorphin Release:**

- o *TENS therapy encourages the release of endorphins, the body's natural painkillers.*
- o *Endorphins help alleviate pain and create a sense of well-being, contributing to overall pain relief during menstruation.*

✓ **Muscle Relaxation:**

- o *TENS devices can promote muscle relaxation, reducing tension in the pelvic area and easing the cramping associated with menstruation.*

Effectiveness of TENS for Menstrual Pain:

Numerous studies and clinical trials have explored the effectiveness of TENS therapy for menstrual pain, with many demonstrating positive outcomes. TENS has been found to significantly reduce pain intensity and improve overall comfort during menstruation. However, individual responses to TENS may vary, and it may not be equally effective for everyone.

Considerations for Choosing a TENS Device:

Adjustable Settings:

- o *Look for a TENS device with adjustable settings for intensity, frequency, and duration to customize the therapy to your comfort level.*

Ease of Use:

- Consider devices with user-friendly interfaces and clear instructions for easy and effective use.

Portability:

- Depending on your lifestyle, you may prefer a compact, portable TENS device that allows you to move freely during use.

Battery Life:

- Check the battery life of the device, especially if you plan to use it for extended periods.

Additional Features:

- Some TENS devices come with additional features such as heat therapy or pre-set programs designed for menstrual pain relief.

Conclusion:

TENS devices offer a non-invasive and drug-free solution for managing menstrual pain, providing relief through the disruption of pain signals, the release of endorphins, and muscle relaxation. With various types of devices available, including traditional TENS units, wearable devices, and those specifically designed for menstrual pain, individuals have options to suit their preferences and lifestyle. Before incorporating TENS therapy into your menstrual pain management routine, it's advisable to consult with a healthcare professional, especially if you have underlying health conditions. Embrace the potential of TENS technology to empower yourself with a personalized and effective approach to menstrual pain relief.

Harmonizing Menstrual Health: Exploring Sound Therapy and Frequencies for Alleviating Menstrual Pain

Menstrual pain, also known as dysmenorrhea, affects millions of women worldwide, impacting their quality of life and productivity. While conventional methods such as pain relievers and heat therapy provide relief for some, an emerging field gaining attention is sound therapy. This holistic approach leverages the power of various frequencies and vibrations to potentially alleviate menstrual pain. In this book, we will delve into the different types of sound therapy and frequencies applied for treating menstrual pain.

Types of Sound Therapy:

❖ **Binaural Beats:**

  ○ *Binaural beats involve playing two slightly different frequencies in each ear, creating a perceived third frequency. This process is believed to influence brainwave patterns and induce a state of relaxation.*

- o *For menstrual pain relief, frequencies in the delta and theta range (0.5 to 8 Hz) are commonly explored, promoting deep relaxation and potentially reducing pain perception.*
- ❖ **Tuning Fork Therapy:**
  - o *Tuning forks are metal instruments that produce a specific sound frequency when struck. When applied to specific points on the body, they may help balance energy and promote healing.*
  - o *Certain frequencies, such as the Solfeggio frequencies (e.g., 174 Hz and 528 Hz), are thought to have healing properties and may be applied during tuning fork therapy for menstrual pain.*
- ❖ **Crystal Singing Bowls:**
  - o *Crystal singing bowls emit pure tones when struck or rubbed with a mallet. Each bowl is tuned to a specific frequency associated with a chakra or healing property.*
  - o *Bowls tuned to frequencies related to the sacral chakra (around 210 Hz) may be used to target the reproductive organs, potentially providing relief from menstrual pain.*
- ❖ **Gong Bath Therapy:**
  - o *Gong baths involve the use of gongs, large metal instruments that produce a wide range of frequencies and harmonics. The vibrations from*

gongs are believed to impact the body at a cellular level.

o   *Specific gong frequencies, such as the Earth Gong tuned to the Schumann Resonance (around 7.83 Hz), may be explored for their potential to promote relaxation and reduce menstrual pain.*

Scientific Basis:

While the scientific understanding of sound therapy's effectiveness for menstrual pain is still in its infancy, some studies suggest a link between sound vibrations and pain perception. For instance, research indicates that exposure to certain frequencies can modulate the autonomic nervous system and influence pain thresholds.

Practical Applications:

Personalized Sound Sessions: *Women experiencing menstrual pain can explore personalized sound therapy sessions tailored to their preferences. This may involve using binaural beats, tuning forks, or singing bowls with frequencies believed to alleviate pain.*

Incorporating Sound into Wellness Routines: *Integrating sound therapy into wellness routines, such as meditation or yoga, may offer a holistic approach to managing menstrual pain. Practices like sound meditation with gongs or singing bowls can create a calming environment.*

Consultation with Sound Therapists: *Seeking guidance from certified sound therapists can provide individuals with tailored approaches to address menstrual pain. These professionals can create targeted sound therapy sessions based on an individual's specific needs and preferences.*

Conclusion:

Sound therapy and frequencies present a fascinating avenue for exploring alternative methods to alleviate menstrual pain. While more research is needed to establish the scientific basis and efficacy of these practices, anecdotal evidence and preliminary studies suggest the potential for positive outcomes. As with any holistic approach, individuals should consult healthcare professionals and experienced sound therapists to determine the most suitable and safe practices for managing menstrual pain. As our understanding of the connection between sound and well-being evolves, sound therapy may become an integral part of holistic menstrual health management.

Mindful Relief: Harnessing the Power of Mindfulness Techniques for Menstrual Pain

In recent years, mindfulness techniques have gained recognition for their potential in managing various health issues, including menstrual pain. In this book, we will explore how mindfulness techniques work and provide practical insights on applying them to alleviate menstrual discomfort.

How Mindfulness Techniques Work:

Mindfulness, rooted in ancient contemplative practices, involves paying attention to the present moment without judgment. Mindfulness techniques work for menstrual pain through several mechanisms:

- ✓ **Pain Perception Alteration:** *Mindfulness practices, such as mindful breathing and body scan meditations, can alter the perception of pain. By fostering a non-judgmental awareness of sensations, individuals may experience a shift in how they relate to and experience menstrual discomfort.*

- ✓ **Stress Reduction:** *Menstrual pain can be exacerbated by stress, which influences hormonal and inflammatory responses. Mindfulness techniques,* *including meditation and deep breathing, are known to activate the body's relaxation response, reducing stress levels and potentially mitigating pain.*

✓ **Cognitive Reappraisal:** *Mindfulness encourages cognitive reappraisal, wherein individuals develop a more balanced and accepting perspective toward their pain. This shift in mindset can lead to a decrease in the emotional impact of menstrual pain.*

Practical Application of Mindfulness Techniques:

❖ **Mindful Breathing:**
  o *Find a quiet space and sit or lie down comfortably.*
  o *Focus your attention on your breath, observing the inhalation and exhalation.*
  o *If your mind wanders, gently bring it back to the breath.*
  o *Practice mindful breathing for 5-10 minutes, especially during the onset of menstrual pain.*

❖ **Body Scan Meditation:**
  o *Lie down in a comfortable position.*
  o *Bring your attention to different parts of your body, starting from your toes and moving up to the head.*
  o *Notice any sensations without judgment. If you encounter tension or discomfort, breathe into that area and release tension as you exhale.*

- o *This practice promotes relaxation and awareness of bodily sensations.*
- ❖ **Mindful Movement:**
  - o *Engage in gentle movement practices like yoga or tai chi.*
  - o *Pay attention to the sensations in your body as you move through different postures.*
  - o *Mindful movement can enhance flexibility, reduce muscle tension, and promote overall well-being.*
- ❖ **Mindfulness-Based Stress Reduction (MBSR):**
  - o *Consider enrolling in a mindfulness-based stress reduction program.*
  - o *MBSR combines meditation, yoga, and awareness practices, offering a structured approach to integrating mindfulness into daily life.*
- ❖ **Mindful Self-Compassion:**
  - o *Cultivate self-compassion by acknowledging and validating your experience of pain.*
  - o *Treat yourself with kindness and understanding, recognizing that discomfort is a part of the natural menstrual cycle.*

Incorporating Mindfulness into Daily Life:

Consistent Practice: *Consistency is key to reaping the benefits of mindfulness. Establish a regular practice, even if it's just a few minutes each day, to build mindfulness skills gradually.*

Integrate Mindfulness into Activities: *Apply mindfulness techniques during routine activities such as eating, walking, or even washing dishes. This helps in cultivating a mindful presence throughout the day.*

Mindfulness Apps: *Explore mindfulness apps that offer guided meditations and exercises specifically designed for managing pain and stress. These can be valuable tools for both beginners and experienced practitioners.*

Conclusion:

Mindfulness techniques provide a promising and accessible avenue for managing menstrual pain. By cultivating awareness, reducing stress, and fostering a compassionate attitude towards one's own experience, individuals can empower themselves to navigate menstrual discomfort with a mindful approach. As mindfulness continues to gain recognition in the realm of holistic health, its integration into the management of menstrual pain offers a holistic and empowering alternative for those seeking relief.

The Power Within: Meditation as a Holistic Treatment for Menstrual Pain Relief and Prevention

Menstrual pain affects countless women each month, leaving them searching for natural and effective remedies. While various approaches exist, meditation has gained recognition as a powerful tool in providing relief and preventing menstrual discomfort. Meditation, an ancient practice that cultivates mindfulness and inner peace, has emerged as a potent holistic approach for alleviating menstrual pain. By tapping into the mind-body connection, meditation targets the underlying causes of the pain, providing both immediate relief and long-term benefits.

How Meditation Works for Menstrual Pain Relief

- ✓ **Increasing Mindfulness:** *Meditation encourages focused attention and awareness of the present moment. By practicing mindfulness during menstruation, you develop a non-judgmental awareness of your body's sensations, effectively reducing pain perception.*

✓ **Stress Reduction:** *Stress exacerbates menstrual pain by constricting muscles and increasing inflammation. Meditation promotes relaxation by activating the body's relaxation response and reducing stress hormones. This, in turn, leads to a reduction in pain intensity.*

✓ **Promoting Hormonal Balance:** *Meditation has been found to help regulate hormone levels in the body. Balanced hormones play a crucial role in managing menstrual pain and promoting overall menstrual health.*

✓ **Enhancing Blood Flow:** *Deep breathing during meditation increases oxygen levels in the body, promoting efficient blood flow. This increased circulation helps relieve cramps and reduces pain and discomfort.*

✓ **Positive Emotional States:** *Regular meditation has been shown to enhance positive emotions and improve overall mood. By cultivating a positive mental state during menstruation, you can better manage emotional fluctuations associated with the menstrual cycle.*

Immediate Pain Relief through Meditation

To experience immediate relief from menstrual pain through meditation, follow these steps:

- ❖ **Find a Quiet and Comfortable Space:** *Choose a calm and peaceful environment where you can sit or lie comfortably without interruption.*

- ❖ **Assume a Comfortable Posture:** *Find a sitting or lying position that supports the natural curves of your spine. You can sit cross-legged on a cushion or lie down with a pillow to support your head and neck.*

- ❖ **Focus on Your Breath:** *Close your eyes and bring your attention to your breath. Notice the rhythm, depth, and sensation of each inhale and exhale.*

- ❖ **Scan Your Body:** *Gradually bring your attention to different parts of your body, starting from your toes and working your way up. Observe any sensations, tension, or pain in each area without judgment.*

- ❖ **Breathe Into the Pain:** *As you notice pain or discomfort, imagine sending your breath to that area. Visualize your breath soothing and healing the pain with each inhale and exhale.*

- ❖ **Maintain Awareness without Resistance:** *Allow any sensations or emotions to arise without resisting or fighting them. Simply observe and acknowledge them with compassionate awareness.*

- ❖ **End with Gratitude:** *Conclude your meditation session by expressing gratitude for your body and its ability to heal. Take a moment to appreciate the time you set aside for self-care and healing.*

Long-Term Pain Prevention with Meditation

To incorporate meditation as a preventive measure against menstrual pain, consider the following practices:

- ❖ **Regular Meditation Practice:** *Aim to meditate daily, even during non-menstrual times. Consistency is key to reaping the long-term benefits of meditation, including hormone balance and stress reduction.*

- ❖ **Menstrual-Specific Meditations:** *Explore guided meditations tailored specifically for menstrual pain relief and prevention. These specialized meditations may include affirmations, visualizations, or targeted body scans.*

- ❖ **Body Awareness Outside Menstruation:** *Cultivate body awareness and practice mindfulness outside of your menstrual cycle. By paying attention to your body's needs and signals, you can better address imbalances before they escalate into menstrual pain.*

- ❖ **Combine with Gentle Exercise:** *Incorporate gentle exercises like yoga or walking into your routine along with meditation. These activities can support overall well-being and further alleviate menstrual pain.*

- ❖ **Seek Professional Guidance:** *Consider seeking guidance from a meditation teacher or therapist who specializes in women's health. They can provide personalized support and guidance on incorporating meditation into your pain prevention regimen.*

Conclusion

Meditation offers a natural and empowering approach to managing menstrual pain, providing immediate relief, and preventing recurring discomfort. By cultivating mindfulness, reducing stress, promoting hormone balance, and enhancing blood flow, meditation taps into the innate intelligence and healing potential of your body. Through consistent practice and a compassionate mindset, you can harness the power within, relieving menstrual pain, and embracing a harmonious and balanced menstrual cycle. Begin your meditation journey today and unlock the transformative path to menstrual pain relief and prevention.

Tranquil Waves: Exploring Hypnotherapy as a Holistic Approach for Menstrual Pain Relief

Hypnotherapy, a form of guided meditation and focused concentration, is gaining recognition as an alternative approach to managing various health issues, including menstrual pain. Hypnotherapy involves inducing a state of deep relaxation and heightened focus, allowing individuals to access their subconscious mind. Contrary to popular misconceptions, individuals under hypnosis remain in control and aware of their surroundings.

Hypnotherapy for menstrual pain relief typically follows these principles:

- ❖ **Relaxation Techniques:** *The hypnotherapist guides the individual into a deeply relaxed state, often beginning with controlled breathing and progressive muscle relaxation. This relaxation helps alleviate stress and tension associated with menstrual pain.*
- ❖ **Visualization:** *Visualization is a key component of hypnotherapy. Individuals are encouraged to imagine*

calming scenes or scenarios, fostering a positive and serene mental environment. This can redirect focus away from pain sensations.

❖ **Suggestion Therapy:** *During hypnosis, the therapist may introduce positive suggestions related to pain reduction and comfort. These suggestions aim to influence the subconscious mind and alter the perception of menstrual pain.*

❖ **Mind-Body Connection:** *Hypnotherapy emphasizes the connection between the mind and body. By addressing psychological factors contributing to pain, such as stress or anxiety, individuals may experience a reduction in the intensity of menstrual discomfort.*

How Hypnotherapy Helps with Menstrual Pain:

✓ **Pain Perception Modification:** *Hypnotherapy has been shown to alter the perception of pain. By guiding individuals to focus their attention away from discomfort and encouraging positive mental imagery, hypnotherapy may help reduce the perceived intensity of menstrual pain.*

✓ **Stress Reduction:** *Stress and anxiety can exacerbate menstrual pain. Hypnotherapy induces a state of deep relaxation, triggering the release of endorphins (natural painkillers) and reducing stress hormones. This can create a more favorable environment for pain relief.*

✓ **Muscle Relaxation:** *Hypnotherapy often includes techniques for progressive muscle relaxation, helping to release tension in the pelvic and abdominal muscles. This can contribute to a decrease in cramping associated with menstrual pain.*

✓ **Addressing Emotional Factors:** *Emotional factors, such as fear or apprehension related to menstrual pain, can contribute to increased discomfort. Hypnotherapy addresses these emotional aspects, fostering a more positive mindset and reducing the emotional impact of pain.*

Applying Hypnotherapy for Menstrual Pain Relief:

❖ **Professional Hypnotherapy Sessions:**
  - *Seek out a qualified hypnotherapist with experience in pain management or women's health. Professional sessions can be tailored to individual needs and provide a guided and structured approach to hypnotherapy.*

❖ **Self-Hypnosis Techniques:**
  - *Learn self-hypnosis techniques through guided recordings or by working with a hypnotherapist. This empowers individuals to practice hypnotherapy independently, especially during menstrual pain episodes.*

❖ **Consistent Practice:**

o   *Consistency is key with hypnotherapy. Regular practice, whether through professional sessions or self-hypnosis, can enhance the effectiveness of the approach over time.*

❖ **Combination with Other Techniques:**

o   *Consider combining hypnotherapy with other holistic approaches such as mindfulness, relaxation exercises, or even conventional treatments for a comprehensive approach to menstrual pain relief.*

Conclusion:

Hypnotherapy, with its focus on the mind-body connection, offers a unique and potentially effective approach to alleviating menstrual pain. By tapping into the subconscious mind and addressing psychological factors, individuals may find relief from the discomfort associated with menstruation. As research in mind-body therapies continues to evolve, hypnotherapy stands as an intriguing avenue for those seeking a holistic and empowering approach to menstrual health.

Closing

Finally Finding Relief: Embracing Healing through Natural and Holistic Remedies for Menstrual Pain

As we reach the end of this enlightening journey through the intricacies of menstrual pain, it is only fitting to close our book by opening the doors to a world of all-natural and holistic treatments.

Gone are the days of relying solely on medications with potential side effects. It is time to unveil a treasure trove of gentle yet effective approaches to alleviating menstrual pain. So, embark on this final voyage with a sense of excitement and curiosity. As you turn the pages, embrace the power of nature. Embrace the power of healing. Your journey begins now.

References

In addition to the references listed here, I also discussed mouth-to-mouth reviews, traditional remedies, and other non-scientific information in this book.

To help my daughter find relief from terrible pain, I collected information over a long period of time and used many different resources.

Having said that, here is a list of some scientific studies on treatments and remedies in the book that can be found in the book:

Por, C., Rajagopal, M., Akowuah, G., Chinnappan, S., & Abdullah, N. (2022). Treatment of primary dysmenorrhea affecting menstruating women using herbs: a review.

Rahnama P, Montazeri A, Vaezi M, et al. A randomized double-blind placebo-controlled trial investigating the effects of ginger extract on dysmenorrhea:
https://pubmed.ncbi.nlm.nih.gov/19216634/Ginger

Sharifi-Rad M, Varoni EM, Iriti M, et al (Khan et al., 2021). A systematic review of the pharmacological effects of chamomile:
https://pubmed.ncbi.nlm.nih.gov/29595380/

McKay DL, Blumberg JB. A review of the bioactivity and potential health benefits of peppermint tea:
https://pubmed.ncbi.nlm.nih.nih.gov/16767798/

Khayat S, Fanaei H, Kheirkhah M, et al. Effect of treatment with ginger on the severity of primary dysmenorrhea is compared to mefenamic acid: https://pubmed.ncbi.nlm.nih.gov/22784340/

Latiff LA, Parhizkar S, Dollah MA, et al (Rahnama et al., 2012). A systematic review on the efficacy and safety of Foeniculum vulgare (fennel) in primary dysmenorrhea: https://pubmed.ncbi.nlm.nih.gov/27871224/

Agustina, V., Khaerunnisa, S., & Dwiningsih, S. (2023). Comparison of the potencies of ginger (zingiber officinale) and fennel (foeniculum vulgare) in ameliorating dysmenorrhea pain: a systematic review

Borrelli F, Ernst E. Alternative and complementary therapies fordysmenorrhea: a systematic review of randomized controlled trials.https://pubmed.ncbi.nlm.nih.gov/16459547/

Santanam N, Klein CB. A review of botanicals commonly used in the treatment of menopause symptoms

Sharifi-Rad J, Salehi B, Stojanović-Radić Z, et al. Antioxidant and anti-inflammatory activities of essential oils from Acacia species

Chemat F, Khan MK, Bekhechi C, et al. A review on the phytochemistry, traditional uses and pharmacological activities of Acacia species

Bent S, Padula A, Moore D, Patterson M, Mehling W. Valerian for Sleep: A systematic review and meta-analysis of randomized controlled trials

Jaafarpour, M., Hatefi, M., Najafi, F., Khajavikhan, J., & Khani, A. (2015). The effect of cinnamon on menstrual bleeding and systemic symptoms with primary dysmenorrhea

Xu, Y., Yang, Q., & Wang, X. (2020). Efficacy of herbal medicine (cinnamon/fennel/ginger) for primary dysmenorrhea: a systematic review and meta-analysis of randomized controlled trials

Manivannan Rajamanickam, Aeganathan Rajamanickam: Analgesic and anti-inflammatory activity of the extracts from Cyperus rotundus Linn rhizomes

Shrivastav, S., Tyagi, R., Cosnier, S., & Jha, S. (2022). The effectiveness of curcumin on dysmenorrhea.

Maia, H., Haddad, C., & Casoy, J. (2014). The effect of pycnogenol on patients with dysmenorrhea using low-dose oral contraceptives

Javaid, T., Mahmood, S., Saeed, W., & Alam, M. (2019). Black cumin (nigella sativa l.): auspicious natural therapy for extensive range of diseases

Su, S., Wang, T., Duan, J., Zhou, W., Hua, Y., Tang, Y., ... & Qian, D. (2011). Anti-inflammatory and analgesic activity of different extracts of commiphora myrrha.

Chen, Y., Chiang, Y., Lin, Y., Huang, K., Chen, H., Hamdy, N., ... & Hsia, S. (2023). Effect of vitamin d supplementation on primary dysmenorrhea: a systematic review and meta-analysis of randomized clinical trials

Chen, R., Moriya, J., & Yamakawa, J.. Chinese herbal medicine for dysmenorrhea

Su, K., Su, S., Ko, C., Cheng, Y., Huang, S., & Chao, J. (2021). Ethnopharmacological survey of traditional chinese medicine pharmacy prescriptions for dysmenorrhea.

Landaeta-Herrera, A., & Artiaga-Perfetti, L.. Ethnobotanical knowledge and natural remedies for dysmenorrhea in South America

Obodozie, I., Okoduwa, S. I., & Osamuyi, O. I.. Ethnobotanical knowledge and medicinal plants used in the treatment of dysmenorrhea in different regions of Africa

Soltanifard, R. ., Shahsavari, S. ., Shakib, P. ., & Abbaszadeh, S. . Phytotherapy and Medicinal Plants in the Treatment of Dysmenorrhea: A Systematic Review Study in Iranian Ethnobotanical Documents.

Qorbanalipour, K., Ghaderi, F., & Jafarabadi, M. (2018). Comparison of the effects of acupressure and electroacupuncture in primary dysmenorrhea: a randomized controlled trial.

Chien, T., Huang, Y., Kuo, C., Cho, Y., Chen, H., Chu, C., ... & Cheng, T. (2020). Do different doses of acupuncture matter on autonomic nervous activity and symptom management in dysmenorrhea?

Sholihah, N. and Azizah, I. (2020). The effect of effleurage massage on primary dysmenorrhea in female adolescent students.

Djupri, D., Manggabarani, S., Irawati, H., & Said, I. (2022). The effect of pelvic rocking exercise and buteyko exercise on reducing primary dysmenorrhea pain levels.

Liu, Y., Yang, L., Yan, B., Jiang, H., Zhao, J., Cao, J., ... & Wang, F. (2021). The effectiveness of acupoint application of traditional chinese medicine in treating primary dysmenorrhea

Sergun, V., Gorbushina, I., Valentina, B., Poznyakovsky, V., Tokhiriyon, B., & Lapina, V. (2022). The use of the new dietary supplement with lake salts in treating primary dysmenorrhea

Heat: Udi, S. and Salamah, U. (2023). Efektivitas pemberian hot herbal compress untuk meredakan dismenore pada remaja putri di smk kesehatan prima indonesia

Ayurveda: nain, O. and Kumar, P. (2023). Critical review on kashtartava (dysmenorrhea-menstrual pain) and its ayurvedic management

Jain, A., Meena, N., & Khathuria, D. (2021). Conceptual study of kashtartavin ayurveda w.s.r. to dysmenorrhoea: literary review.

Yuliani, E. (2023). The effect of dark chocolate on the intensity of primary dysmenorrhea pain in female students.

Sari, K., Nasifah, I., & Trisna, A. (2018). Pengaruh senam yoga terhadap nyeri haid remaja putri. Jurnal Kebidanan

Weisberg, M. Chronic pelvic pain and hypnosis.

Belcaro G,1 Cornelli U,2 Hernández Santos JR3. Treatment of Dysmenorrhea with Physiological Modulators (A28): A Registry Study*

Idauli Simbolon, Florida Hutabarat, Nilawati Soputri, Denny Ricky, Ayu Nathania, Monica Rahel Sabattini, IMPLEMENTATION OF DEEP BREATHING RELAXATION, MUSIC THERAPY, AND EFFLUERAGE MASSAGE THERAPY TO DECREASE PAIN SCALE OF DYSMENORHEA AMONG COLLEGE STUDENTS

JENNINGS C. LITZENBERG, B.S., M.D. THE USE OF BENZYL BENZOATE IN DYSMENORRHEA

Liu, C., Xie, J., Wang, L., Zheng, Y., Ma, Z., Yang, H., ... & Liu, J. (2011). Immediate analgesia effect of single point acupuncture in primary dysmenorrhea: a randomized controlled trial